TRANSESOPHAGEAL ECHOCARDIOGRAPHY

DEVELOPMENTS IN CRITICAL CARE MEDICINE AND ANESTHESIOLOGY

Prakash, O. (ed.): Applied Physiology in Clinical Respiratory Care. 1982. ISBN 90-247-2662-X.

McGeown, Mary G.: Clinical Management of Electrolyte Disorders. 1983. ISBN 0-89838-559-8.

Scheck, P.A., Sjöstrand, U.H., and Smith, R.B. (eds.): Perspectives in High Frequency Ventilation. 1983. ISBN 0-89838-571-7.

Stanley, T.H., and Petty, W.C. (eds.): New Anesthetic Agents, Devices and Monitoring Techniques. 1983. ISBN 0-89838-566-0.

Prakash, O. (ed.): Computing in Anesthesia and Intensive Care. 1983. ISBN 0-89838-602-0.

Stanley, T.H., and Petty, W.C. (eds.): Anesthesia and the Cardiovascular System. 1984. ISBN 0-89838-626-8.

Van Kleef, J.W., Burm, A.G.L., and Spierdijk, J. (eds.): Current Concepts in Regional Anaesthesia. 1984. ISBN 0-89838-644-6.

Prakash, O. (ed.): Critical Care of the Child. 1984. ISBN 0-89838-661-6.

Stanley, T.H., and Petty, W.C. (eds.): Anesthesiology: Today and Tomorrow. 1985. ISBN 0-89838-705-1.

Rahn, H., and Prakash, O. (eds.): Acid-base Regulation and Body Temperature. 1985. ISBN 0-89838-708-6.

Stanley, T.H., and Petty, W.C. (eds.): Anesthesiology 1986. ISBN 0-89838-779-5.

de Lange, S., Hennis, P.J., and Kettler, D. (eds.): Cardiac Anaesthesia: Problems and Innovations. 1986. ISBN 0-89838-794-9.

deBruijn, N.P., and Clements, F.M.: Transesophageal Echocardiography. 1987. ISBN 0-89838-821-X.

Graybar, G.B., and Bready, L.L. (eds.): Anesthesia for Renal Transplantation. 1987. ISBN 0-89838-837-6.

Stanley, T.H., and Petty, W.E. (eds.): Anesthesia, the Heart, and the Vascular System. 1987. ISBN 0-89838-851-1.

TRANSESOPHAGEAL ECHOCARDIOGRAPHY

NORBERT P. DE BRUIJN, M.D.
Associate Professor
Department of Anesthesiology and Surgery
Duke University
Durham, North Carolina

FIONA M. CLEMENTS, M.D.
Assistant Professor
Department of Anesthesiology
Duke University
Durham, North Carolina

with a contribution by

RUSSELL HILL, M.D.
Fellow, Division of Cardiothoracic Anesthesia
Duke University Medical Center
Durham, North Carolina

MARTINUS NIJHOFF PUBLISHING
A MEMBER OF THE KLUWER ACADEMIC PUBLISHERS GROUP
BOSTON/DORDRECHT/LANCASTER

Distributors

for the United States and Canada: Kluwer Academic Publishers, 101 Philip Drive,
Norwell, MA 02061, USA

for the UK and Ireland: Kluwer Academic Publishers, MTP Press Limited, Falcon
House, Queen Square, Lancaster LA1 1RN, UK

for all other countries: Kluwer Academic Publishers Group, Distribution Centre,
P.O. Box 322, 3300 AH Dordrecht, The Netherlands

Library of Congress Cataloging-in-Publication Data

Transesophageal echocardiography.

(Developments in critical care medicine and anesthesiology; 13)
Includes bibliographies and index.
1. Heart—Diseases—Diagnosis. 2. Transesophageal echocardiography.
I. DeBruijn, Norbert P. II. Clements, Fiona M. III. Hill, Russell, 1955-   .
IV. Series: Developments in critical care medicine and anaesthesiology; 13. [DNLM:
1. Echocardiography. 2. Ultrasonic Diagnosis. WG 141.5.E2 T772]
RC683.5.T83T73 1986   616.1'207'543   86-17959
ISBN-13: 978-1-4612-9206-7   e-ISBN-13: 978-1-4613-2025-8
DOI: 10.1007/978-1-4613-2025-8

CONTENTS

FOREWORD

Almost every effort in the care of patients with heart disease begins with some description of disordered physiologic performance or morphologic anatomy. Since the early work of Edler and Hertz in 1954, echocardiographic methods have grown in importance and reliability for the diagnosis of many cardiac disorders.

The placement of a maneuverable transducer on the tip of a modified endoscope is the result of relatively recent technologic advances. The transesophageal approach is now a reality for obtaining new information from ultra-sonic images of a beating human heart.

Since images obtained by transesophageal echocardiography are uniformly of excellent quality, it extends the diagnostic potential of echocardiography to the patient who is difficult to image from the conventional chest wall approach.

More importantly, transesophageal echocardiography provides a means to acquire useful information in new situations, such as the operating room. When this imaging modality is brought to patients undergoing surgical procedures, surgeons and anesthesiologists have a ready means for assessing cardiac performance during anesthesia, directing various surgical approaches and immediately evaluating the results of surgical repair.

Transesophageal echocardiographic techniques represent a major advance in the care of patients with cardiovascular disease. Never before has there been a means to acquire such important information about the heart during an operative intervention. New questions are being asked and new answers are at hand.

This book by Drs. de Bruijn and Clements captures these exciting new developments as they explain the fundamentals and current and future applications of transesophageal echocardiography. The authors provide a timely definition of the practice through their insights and experiences. Serious students or practitioners of the healing arts with interest in cardiovascular disease will find this volume of extraordinary value.

Echocardiographic practice has generally fallen within the domain of cardiologists, internists, or radiologists. The authors amply demonstrate that others with similar interest and enthusiasm expand our knowledge of cardiac anatomy and function and ultimately improve our care of patients. Although the impact of their efforts, and those of their colleagues involved in similar pursuits, is yet to be fully realized, they are likely to redefine the requisite fund of knowledge and skills necessary for the practice of cardiovascular anesthesiology in the future.

Joseph Kisslo
Associate Professor
of Medicine

PREFACE

This book, deriving from the experience of anesthesiologists, tends to reflect the use of transesophageal echocardiography as it has become known in the USA. The reader should realize, however, that in Europe the use of transesophageal echocardiography has been almost entirely in the hands of cardiologists. We have tried to present the experiences of both specialists in this work and hope that both groups will find it of interest. We believe that the full potential of transesophageal echocardiography at an institution can only be realized when cardiologists and anesthesiologists have joint responsibility and interest in its use. Our own endeavors have been strongly supported by Joseph Kisslo, who gave us not only the benefit of his own vast experience in echocardiography, but also provided the administrative leadership necessary to establish the use of transesophageal echocardiography as a clinical service.

We are indebted to a number of other people whose special efforts have facilitated the completion of this manuscript.

Michael Feneley and J.G. Reves provided us with ideas, inspiration, and constructive criticism.

Nancy Henn, with the excellent illustrations, helped us to describe the cardiac anatomy as it is seen with transesophageal echocardiography.

Ann Hogan and Gail Brooks provided considerable patience and understanding along with their secretarial assistance.

Lastly, we would like to thank the Diasonics Corporation, which made a transesophageal imaging system available to us in the first place.

TRANSESOPHAGEAL ECHOCARDIOGRAPHY

1. DEVELOPMENT OF TRANSESOPHAGEAL ECHOCARDIOGRAPHY

Technology using reflected sound waves to localize objects was initially developed for naval sonar but expanded in many directions. The use of ultrasound for imaging dynamic cardiac structures was first introduced in 1954 by Edler and Hertz [1] and has since revolutionized diagnostic approaches to cardiac disease. Ultrasound waves reflected from cardiac surfaces can be presented as dots or moving lines (M-mode echocardiography), but a more understandable representation of the heart is provided when the reflected ultrasound waves are oriented in two dimensions to produce an image resembling a cross section of the heart (2D echocardiography). Transmission of ultrasound into living tissue has proved to be safe, and comfortable for patients; thus since 1954 many refinements have taken place to explore its full potential in clinical and research use. A variety of hand-held transducers capable of emitting and receiving ultrasound have been used by cardiologists. The standard technique requires that the transducer is placed on the skin surface overlying the heart. Since ultrasound frequencies are not transmitted well through air, contact between the skin and the transducer is maintained by the use of a coupling gel applied liberally to the skin. The heart lies at a variable depth within the thorax and thus cardiac imaging is often facilitated by positioning the patient on his left side so that the heart falls against

1

the left anterior chest wall. With all the various improvements in equipment, successful cardiac imaging still requires first of all that the heart lie within the field of view of the ultrasound transducer, and it is essentially this particular aspect of imaging that led to the development of esophageal transducers.

Early on it became clear that patients with barrel chests, chronic obstructive pulmonary disease, or simple obesity were difficult to image with a transducer placed on the chest wall; this was simply because of the amount of tissue intervening between the transducer and the heart. In particular those parts of the heart most distant from the transducer were most difficult to image. There is a finite depth of field for any transducer, representing the distance over which ultrasound waves can be transmitted and received from cardiac structures with sufficient resolution to generate a useful image. For the 10%–30% patients whose anatomy makes conventional transthoracic imaging difficult, the esophagus provides an obvious access with which the transducer can be placed immediately adjacent to the posterior surface of the heart. For this approach to become a practical option, the transducer had to be of a size that could be swallowed fairly easily. Early work with M-mode transesophageal echocardiography was reported in 1976 by Frazin and coworkers [2], using a transducer assembly measuring 19 × 13 × 6 mm attached to a coaxial cable, which allowed some rotational control (figure 1-1).

Image quality compared very well with transthoracic images, and allowed definition of structures poorly seen from the chest wall in certain patients. Although image orientation required some adjustment for the cardiologist, used to imaging from the opposite direction, the technique was found to be fairly simple. This early work pointed out the need for external controls that could be used to direct the ultrasound beam in various planes. Such flexibility was afforded by mounting the ultrasound transducer within a commercially available flexible gastroscope, substituting the electrical wires for the original fiberoptics. This has proved to be a very useful arrangement, offering considerable flexibility for imaging the heart in multiple planes and is a convenient and comfortable instrument for both patient and echocardiographer.

Matsumoto and coworkers [3] reported their experience with this improved transesophageal probe for evaluating left ventricular performance during supine bicycle exercise; their instrument, provided by Aerotech Corporation, measured 24 × 14 × 11 mm at the transducer location and provided images adequate for analysis in exercis-

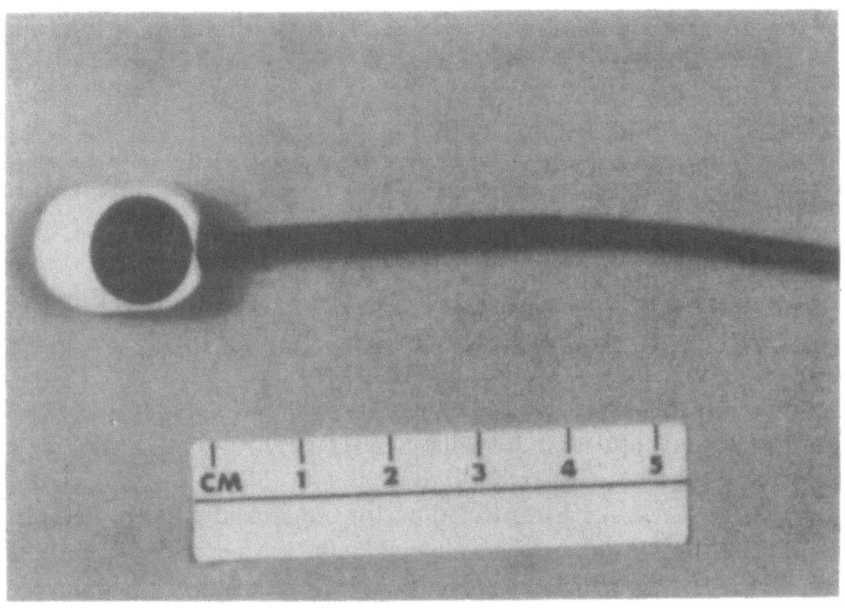

Figure 1-1. Photograph of esophageal transducer. Reproduced with permission from Frazin et al. [2].

ing subjects. Study of dynamic cardiac function during exercise is impaired by chest wall motion and exaggerated lung excursions; transesophageal imaging appeared to offer some advantage over the transthoracic approach for these reasons, but cannot have been altogether comfortable for the subjects.

Matsumoto also used transesophageal M-mode echocardiography in anesthetized patients [4], where problems of patient cooperation and discomfort were obviously eliminated. Images were satisfactory and cardiac output determinations from echo data correlated well with those obtained by thermodilution. Interest in monitoring left ventricular function in anesthetized patients using ultrasound techniques had previously been demonstrated by Barash and coworkers [5], who employed a parasternally placed transducer to obtain M-mode echocardiograms. Similarly, Rathod and coworkers [6] used transthoracic ultrasound techniques to compare the effects of two inhalational anesthetics on cardiac performance. Whereas M-mode echocardiography continues to enjoy widespread use, 2D imaging became available for transthoracic use, and eventually found its way into the esophagus.

2D imaging was accomplished originally with a mechanically

rotated transducer, which scanned an arc at high speed to produce real-time 2D images displayed on a cathode ray tube monitor. This kind of transducer and cable was adapted for transesophageal use and described by Hisanaga and coworkers [7], who evaluated it in 67 patients. Because the transducer was required to rotate mechanically within the esophagus at high speed, it was enclosed within an oil bag to eliminate discomfort and friction in the esophagus. The size of this oil bag could be varied, to a maximum diameter of 15 mm, and the transducer assembly measured 12 × 20 × 6 mm. The cable was encased in a flexible shaft and the arc of transducer rotation was, with this instrument, 360° (figures 1-2 and 1-3).

For transesophageal imaging, mechanically rotated transducers have been largely supplanted by phased array transducers, which were described by Drs. Kisslo, Von Ramm and Thurstone, in 1976 for transthoracic use [8, 9]. Electronically controlled phasing of ultrasound pulses from each of several transducer elements provided an alternative to mechanical rotation of a transducer to generate a two-dimensional image. Phased array transducers became widely employed for conventional transthoracic 2D imaging and it was not long before a phased array transducer was adapted for transesophageal use. Much of the credit for this development must go to Dr. Hanrath's group in Hamburg. In 1982, this group reported their experience with a miniature phased array ultrasound transducer again fitted into a commercially available gastroscope, which they used in 26 awake patients [10]. This instrument measured 35 × 15 × 16 mm and included 32 transducer elements. In contrast to the rotating scanner, this instrument provided a 90% sector scan, with a higher line density and therefore a clearer image. External control of transducer angulation was improved over previous systems, and the assembly was well tolerated by patients. Since the transducer did not rotate or vibrate, there was no need for an oil bag and good contact with the esophageal wall was maintained easily with transducer angulation. These investigators predicted that transesophageal 2D echocardiography would find application for morphological diagnosis of atrial thrombi, atrial septal defects, and mitral valve prolapse, which are particularly well imaged from an esophageal approach, and also for myocardial contraction abnormalities. The ability to monitor cardiac function and detect intracardiac air intraoperatively was clearly attractive and it appeared that there was no risk to patients undergoing this procedure. Later work by Dr. Hanrath's group in association with Dr. Cahalan at UCSF was published in 1985 reporting experi-

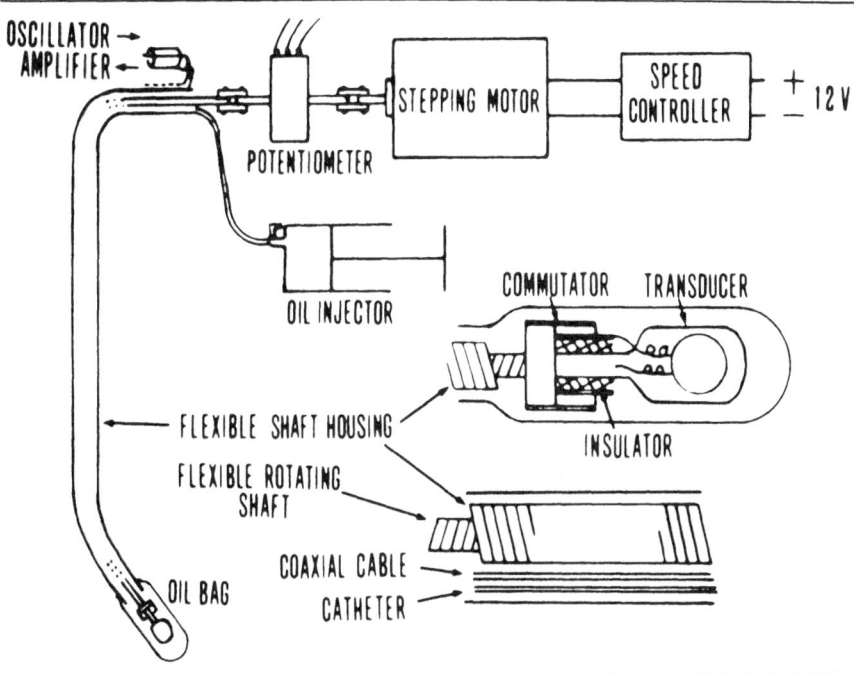

Figure 1-2. Diagrammatic illustration of the transesophageal high-speed rotating scanner. Reproduced with permission from Hisanaga et al. [7].

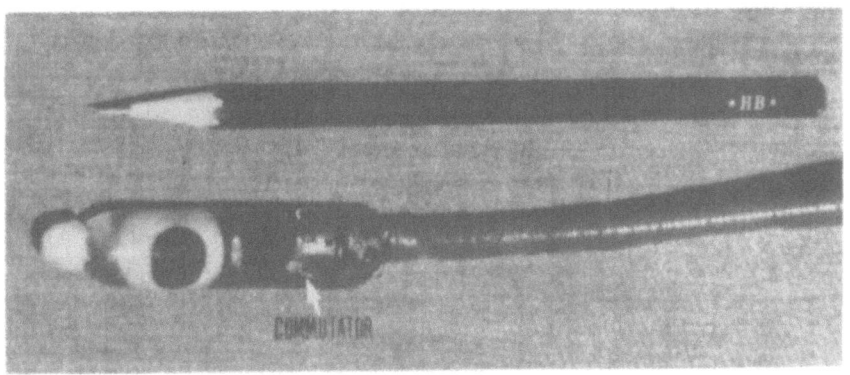

Figure 1-3. Transducer and commutator in oil bag. Sound energy is coupled to and from the transducer through the slip-ring commutator because of the full 360° rotation of the transducer. Reproduced with permission from Hisanaga et al. [7].

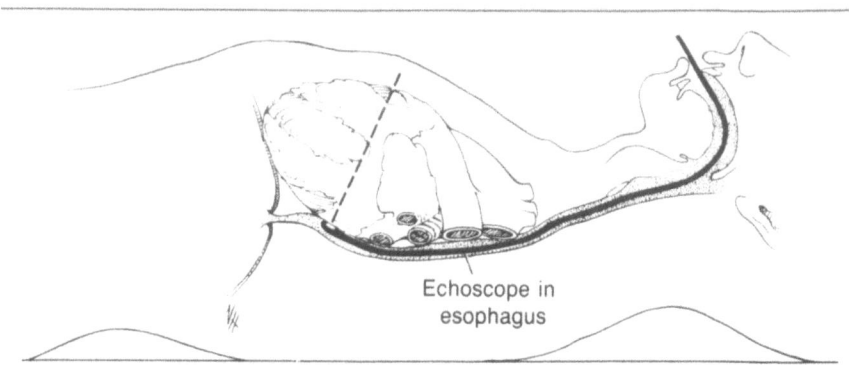

Echoscope in
esophagus

Figure 1-4. Diagram of phased array esophageal transducer in position for cardiac imaging.

ence with transesophageal echocardiography in over 400 patients undergoing elective surgery. High-quality images of the left ventricle suitable for quantitative analysis [11] were obtained in 87% of these patients. In only 5% of patients was image quality totally inadequate. No complications were seen in this group, except for two patients in whom the transducer could not be introduced blindly into the esophagus. Concurrently with this study, numerous investigators have explored the use of transesophageal echocardiography in anesthetized patients, at several centers in the United States.

Since ultrasound waves can be used to measure the velocity of blood flow by the Doppler principle (see chapter 6), the development of ultrasound imaging techniques has been accompanied by Doppler technology. This has been used to evaluate blood flow in the aorta, representing cardiac output, and blood flow through valves and congenital defects for the characterization of valvular heart disease and intracardiac shunts. Transesophageal Doppler was first investigated in 1971 by Side and Gosling, who used Doppler velocity measurements in the thoracic aorta for assessment of cardiac function [12]. Transesophageal pulsed Doppler echocardiography was later reported by Hanrath's group in 1982 and found to be superior to a transthoracic approach for the diagnosis of mild to moderately severe mitral regurgitation [13].

The use of transesophageal ultrasound transducers for cardiac imaging and Doppler flow measurements has therefore been under investigation, mostly by cardiologists, for approximately ten years. For the cardiologist familiar with ultrasound images, transesophageal imaging extends his expertise, provided he invests some time in learning to manipulate the modified flexible gastroscope, and becomes familiar with the altered orientation of images recorded from the esophagus. Since the introduction of the esophageal probe into awake patients requires some topical anesthesia to the pharynx and intravenous sedation, many cardiologists find the procedure too inconvenient to justify the time and effort required. Hanrath's group, for example, has suggested that two months of gastroscopic practice is helpful, and that, with experience, a complete examination from the esophagus then takes approximately 10 min.

Besides cardiologists, it is anesthesiologists who have been interested in transesophageal imaging. The search for better ways to assess cardiac performance intraoperatively has accelerated in recent years as more elderly patients undergo surgery and as the growth of cardiac surgery has expanded. For anesthesiologists, echocardiography provides beat-to-beat information about contractility and preload, which can otherwise only be indirectly assessed by invasive monitoring techniques. Furthermore, it offers, for the first time, information about regional function, providing the most sensitive method yet available to the clinician to detect ischemia (see chapter 4).

With increasing interest in transesophageal echocardiography, several manufacturers have developed esophageal transducers, following the lead of the Diasonics Corporation, which has had one available for several years. The expansion of the echocardiography market into the area of patient monitoring gives us reason to hope that transesophageal imaging systems will become less expensive.

REFERENCES

1. Edler I, Hertz CH: Use of ultrasonic reflectoscope for continuous recording of movement of heart walls. Kung Fysiogr Sallsk Lund Fordhandl 24:40, 1954.
2. Frazin L, Talano JV, Stephanides L, Loeb HS, Kopel L, Gunnar RM: Esophageal echocardiography. Circulation 54:102–108, 1976.
3. Matsumoto M, Hanrath P, Kremer P, Tams C, Langenstein BA, Schlüter M, Weiter R, Bleifeld W: Evaluation of left ventricular performance during supine exercise by transoesophageal M-mode echocardiography in normal subjects. Br Heart J 48:61–66, 1982.
4. Matsumoto M, Oka Y, Strom J, Frishman W, Kadish A, Becker RM, Frater RWM, Sonneblick EH: Application of transesophageal echocardiography to continuous intraoperative monitoring of left ventricular performance. Am J Cardiol 46:95–105, 1980.
5. Barash PG, Glanz S, Katz JD, Taunt K, Talner NS: Ventricular function in children during halothane anesthesia: an echocardiographic evaluation. Anesthesiology 49:79–85, 1978.
6. Rathod R, Jacobs HK, Kramer NE, Rao TLK, Salem MR, Towne WD: Echocar-

diographic assessment of ventricular performance following induction with two anesthetics. Anesthesiology 49:86–90, 1978.

7. Hisanaga K, Hisanaga A, Hibi N, Nishimura K, Kambe T: High speed rotating scanner for transesophageal cross-sectional echocardiography. Am J Cardiol 46:837–842, 1980.

8. Von Ramm OT, Thurstone FL: Cardiac imaging using a phased array ultrasound System. I. System design. Circulation 53:258–262, 1976.

9. Kisslo J, Von Ramm OT, Thurstone FL: Cardiac imaging using a phased array ultrasound system. II. Clinical technique and application. Circulation 53:262–267, 1976.

10. Schlüter M, Langenstein BA, Polster J, Kremer P, Souquet J, Engel S, Hanrath P: Transoesophageal cross-sectional echocardiography with a phased array transducer system: technique and initial clinical results. Br Heart J 48:67–72, 1982.

11. Kremer P, Cahalan M, Beaupre P, Schröder E, Hanrath P, Heinrich H, Ahnefeld FW, Bleifeld W, Hamilton W: Intraoperative Überwachung mittels transoesophagealer zweidimensionaler Echokardiographie. Anaesthesist 34:111–117, 1985.

12. Side CD, Gosling RG: Non-surgical assessment of cardiac function. Nature 232:335–336, 1971.

13. Schlüter M, Langenstein BA, Hanrath P, Kremer P, Bleifeld W: Assessment of tranesophageal pulsed Doppler echocardiography in the detection of mitral regurgitation. Circulation 66:784–789, 1982.

2. PRINCIPLES OF ULTRASOUND

RUSSELL HILL

Effective use of 2D echocardiography requires that the user acquire some understanding of how the images are produced. Although modern technology has resulted in images that quite faithfully represent the structures scanned by the transducer, ultrasound has limitations that should be understood for the correct interpretation of echocardiographic images.

In 1880, the Curie brothers demonstrated that a properly cut piece of quartz develops electric charges on its surface when subjected to a deforming mechanical stress. This is now known as the piezoelectric or pressure electric effect. The voltage developed across a piezoelectric element by a mechanical stress is proportional to the amplitude of the stress. Conversely, the Curies also observed that, when a piezoelectric crystal is placed in an electric field, it is mechanically deformed, and produces ultrasound waves. The transmission and reception of energy, in the form of ultrasound waves, by the piezoelectric elements in the transducer, constitutes the physical basis for ultrasound imaging. Although several natural minerals exhibit the piezoelectric effect, artificial ceramic materials called ferroelectrics are used in most modern ultrasound transducers. The quality of image produced and the depth of field that can be examined are limited significantly by the frequency or wavelength of ultrasound that can be emitted by the

9

transducer. Transducers are commonly described by this standard frequency, e.g., 3.5 MHz, 5 MHz, 10 MHz. The generation of an ultrasound image depends on many properties of wave motion and on the characteristics of the tissue through which the ultrasound waves travel.

PROPERTIES OF WAVE MOTION

Wave motion is a universal phenomenon with which energy is transferred from one point to another. Mechanical waves, of which sound and ultrasound are examples, differ from electromagnetic waves such as light in that they require a physical medium to travel through. Mechanical waves originate in the displacement of a portion of an elastic medium from its normal position. Because of elastic forces on adjacent areas, the disturbance is propagated from the origin throughout the medium. The medium does not move as a whole but its component parts oscillate periodically about their equilibrium position.

Mechanical waves can be classified according to the type of motion exhibited by the particles of matter within their respective media. Transverse waves consist of particles displaced perpendicular to the direction of wave propagation. Waves characterized by particle oscillation parallel to the direction of wave propagation are called longitudinal waves. Sound and ultrasound waves in gaseous and liquid media are examples of longitudinal waves. Figure 2-1 illustrates a continuous train of periodic longitudinal waves that can be considered as a series of compressions and rarefactions. A surface including all points undergoing a similar disturbance at a given instant represents a wave front. If waves are propagated in only one direction, wave fronts are parallel planes. Mechanical waves originating from a point source emanate radially in all three dimensions and their wavefronts are spherical (see figure 2-1).

The velocity of longitudinal mechanical waves through a particular medium depends on the physical properties of that medium. In a gas or liquid:

$$V = \sqrt{B/\rho}$$

where B is the bulk modulus of elasticity and ρ is the density [1]. The velocity of sound or ultrasound in air is 381.3 m/s. In human soft tissue, it is approximately 1540 m/s [2]. The wavelength (λ) is the distance between consecutive points of the wave where the magnitude

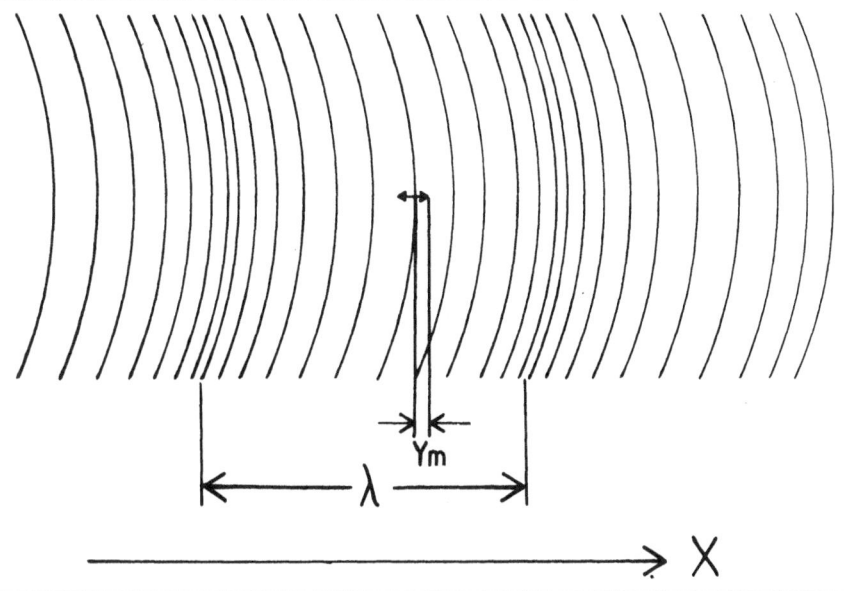

Figure 2-1. λ = wavelength, Y_m = amplitude, and X = direction of wave propagation.

of displacement is identical. The frequency is the number of wave cycles that pass a given point in the medium per unit of time, usually expressed in cycles per second or hertz. Frequency of the wave is determined by the frequency of oscillation of the source. Wavelength and frequency are inversely proportional to each other and related to the velocity by:

$$V = f\lambda$$

Longitudinal mechanical waves are generated over a large range of frequencies, but sound is confined to waves within the frequency range that stimulates the human ear and brain to the sensation of hearing. The audible range is from 20 to 20,000 Hz; ultrasound waves are of frequencies greater than 20,000 Hz, with those frequencies used in echocardiography being in the range of millions of Hz, or megahertz (MHz).

The energy per unit of time, or power, transferred through a medium is called intensity (I) and is expressed in watts per square centimeter. It is sometimes desirable to compare the intensities of two waves. Since the intensities of sound or ultrasound waves vary over many orders of magnitude, it is convenient to measure the logarithm of the ratios of the intensity or amplitude of two waves; the decibel notation is commonly used. The ratio of intensity of two waves in decibels is:

$$dB = 20 \log A_1/A_2 = 10 \log I_1/I_2$$

where A is amplitude and I is intensity [3]. It must be realized that the decibel notation is used only to compare intensity of two waves with each other or with a reference intensity; the decibel is not a measure of absolute power.

Mechanical waves passing through a particular medium act independently of one another. The displacement of any one point at a given time is the vector sum of the displacements resulting from all waves passing through at that time. If two waves are in phase, amplitude is increased; if they are out of phase, they tend to cancel each other out and amplitude is reduced. When a mechanical system is acted on by a wave, it tends to vibrate at the frequency of that wave. If the frequency of the incident wave is close to one of the natural frequencies of oscillation of the system, it vibrates with a relatively large amplitude. This phenomenon is called resonance and natural frequencies of oscillation are called resonant frequencies.

As a wave is propagated from its source through a medium, its intensity is reduced, or attenuated, as a function of the distance it travels. Attenuation is due to divergence of beam width, scattering of wave energy, reflection, and absorption. Absorption is the process that transforms vibrational energy into heat. The amplitude absorption coefficient μ is described by:

$$\mu = -(1/x) \log_e (A_x/A_o)$$

where A_x = amplitude at x centimeters from the source, and A_o = peak amplitude at the source.

The quantity μ is a logarithm of the ratios of two amplitudes very similar to the decibel notation. Multiplying μ by $20 \log_e$ gives the attenuation coefficient (α) in units of dB per centimeter [2]. There is experimental evidence that the attenuation coefficient (α) of ultrasound in most nonbiological fluids is proportional to the square of the frequency. In biological soft tissue, however, α is more closely related to the frequency raised to the first power for ultrasound with frequencies of 0.2–10 MHz [2]. Ultrasound of high frequency is attenuated more severely than low-frequency ultrasound and therefore

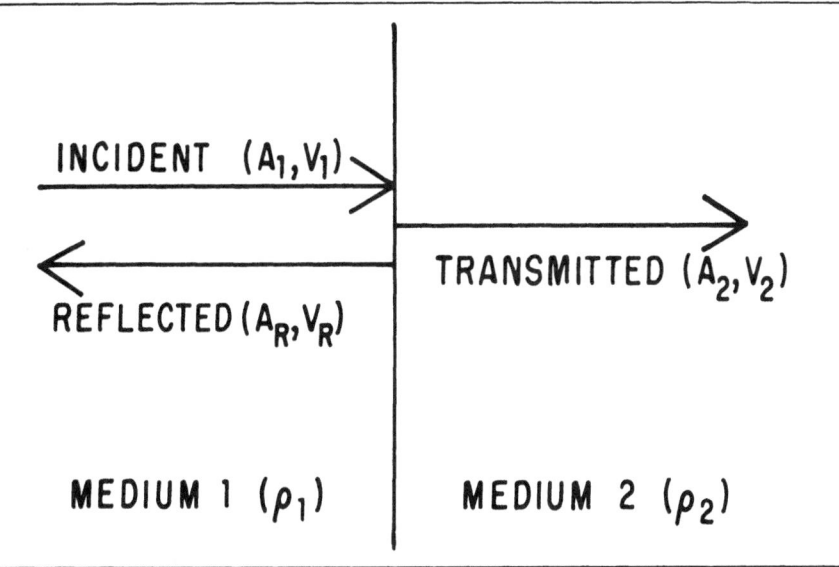

Figure 2-2. A_1, = amplitude of incident wave, A_R = amplitude of reflected wave, A_2 = amplitude of transmitted wave, V_1 = velocity of ultrasound in medium 1, V_2 = velocity of ultrasound in medium 2, $\rho 1$ and $\rho 2$ = densities of mediums 1 and 2, and $V_R = V_1$.

does not penetrate through tissue as far. As a general rule, the attenuation coefficient of ultrasound in soft tissue is approximately 1 dB/cm/MHz [4].

BEHAVIOR OF ULTRASOUND AT BOUNDARIES

In clinical use, ultrasound images are produced by reflected waves or echoes from objects within the field of examination. When an ultrasonic beam meets a boundary between two media with different acoustic properties, part of the beam is reflected and part is transmitted into the second medium. If the dimensions of the boundary are large compared with the wave length of ultrasound, the quantity of energy reflected is proportional to the difference in acoustic impedance of the two media. Acoustic impedance is equal to the product of the density of the medium and the velocity of ultrasound within the medium [5]. The ratio of the amplitude of the reflected wave to the amplitude of the original incident wave is called the amplitude reflection coefficient. Figure 2-2 illustrates an ultrasound wave with amplitude A_1, and velocity V_1, traveling through a medium of density ρ_1, as it strikes a boundary of a second medium of density ρ_2. If the boundary is perpendicular to the incident wave, the amplitude of the reflected wave, A_R, is the product of A_1, and the reflection coefficient [5], R_{12}, expressed as:

$$A_R = A_1 (R_{12}) = A_1 \frac{\rho_1 V_1 - \rho_2 V_2}{\rho_1 V_1 + \rho_2 V_2}$$

The amplitude of the transmitted wave through the second medium (A_2) is expressed by:

$$A_2 = A_1 \frac{2\rho_1 V_1}{\rho_1 V_1 + \rho_2 V_2}$$

The reflected wave returns through the first medium at the same frequency and velocity as the original incident wave.

The directions of reflected and transmitted ultrasound waves follow Snell's Law as do light waves. The angle of reflection equals the angle of incidence as shown in figure 2-3. The angle of a transmitted ultrasound wave is related to the ratio of the velocity of ultrasound within the two media. Fortunately the velocity of ultrasound in different human soft tissues is similar and the angle of transmission is close enough to the angle of incidence that an ultrasound beam is considered to travel in a straight line across boundaries and through different media.

Boundaries that are large with respect to the wavelength of ultrasound and cause reflections that behave as described above are known as specular reflectors and produce specular echoes (figure 2-4a). The quantity of energy reflected back toward the source from a specular reflector depends on the angle of the reflector with respect to the ultrasound beam as well as on the acoustic mismatch across boundaries. As the angle of incidence increases, the portion of energy reflected toward the source is decreased.

In addition to specular reflectors, ultrasound waves may encounter discrete objects or irregularities on large objects that are small relative to the wavelength. These objects or irregularities reflect and scatter ultrasound in all directions (figure 2-4b). The amplitude of scattered echoes is small, but the reception and detection of them is much less angle dependent than specular echoes. The production of scattered echoes enables the reception of echoes from surfaces whose boundaries are not perpendicular to the incident ultrasound beam. From this discussion, it should be clear that a cardiac structure may or may not appear clearly on an ultrasound image, according to its

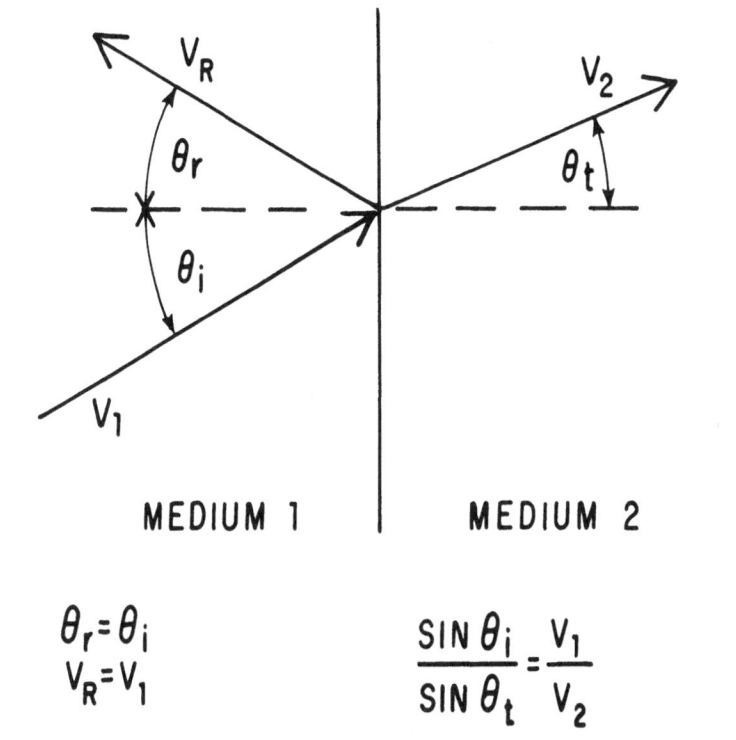

$$\theta_r = \theta_i$$
$$V_R = V_1$$

$$\frac{SIN\ \theta_i}{SIN\ \theta_t} = \frac{V_1}{V_2}$$

Figure 2-3. θ_i = angle of incidence, θ_r = angle of reflection, θ_t = angle of transmission, V_1 = velocity of ultrasound in medium 1, V_2 = velocity of ultrasound in medium 2, and V_R = velocity of reflected ultrasound.

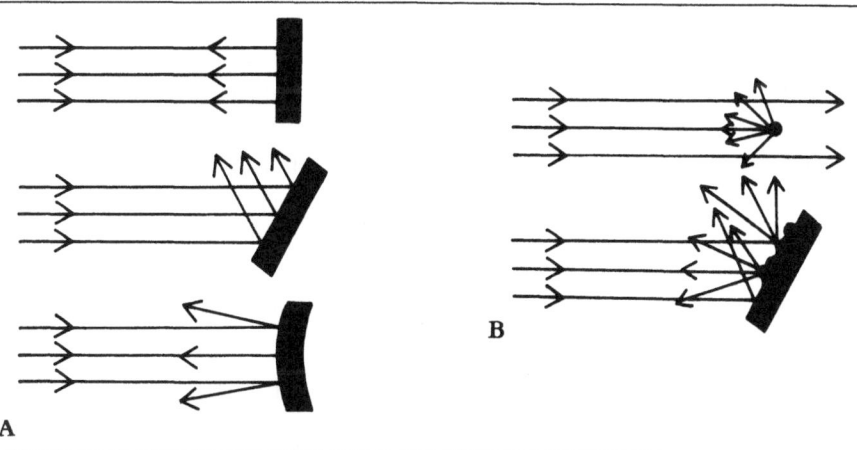

Figure 2-4. (a) Specular echoes. (b) Scattered echoes.

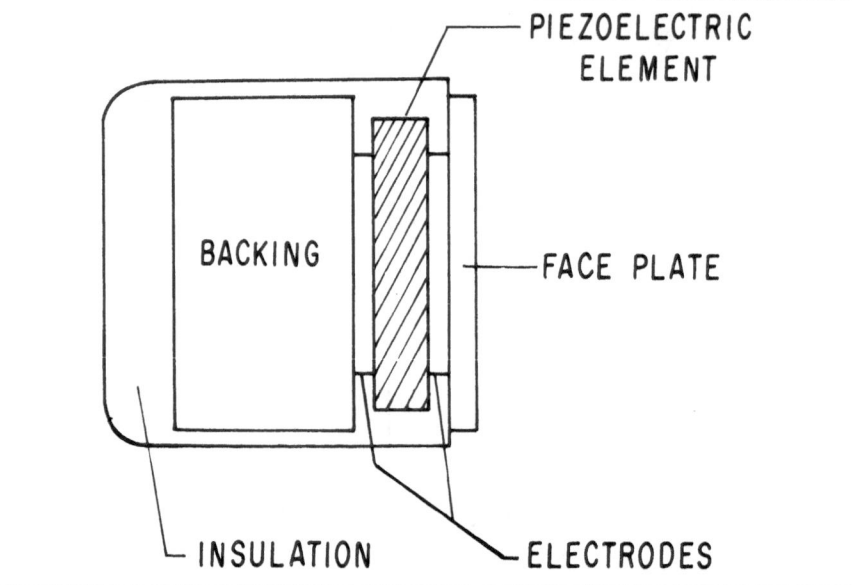

Figure 2-5. Transducer components.

distance from the transducer, and the angle at which the incident ultrasound waves strike it. Structures reflecting specular echoes that are positioned fairly close to the transducer, having borders lying perpendicular to the beam, will be delineated most clearly. Those structures reflecting scattered echoes, oriented parallel to the beam, will be least well defined.

ULTRASOUND BEAMS AND TRANSDUCERS

The effective use of ultrasound in diagnostic echocardiography depends on the generation of a short pulse of ultrasound energy that is propagated in a straight narrow beam. The pulse of ultrasound energy must be reflected by cardiac structures back toward the transducer, converted to electrical energy, and then displayed in some interpretable fashion before the next pulse is generated. The essential components of an ultrasound transducer are shown in figure 2-5. A narrow beam of pulsed ultrasound is generated by a disc of piezoelectric material that is electrically excited by two electrodes on either parallel surface. If an alternating voltage is applied across the piezoelectric element, variations in its thickness occur at the frequency of alternating voltage. Movement of the surfaces of the piezoelectric element produces compressions and rarefactions that are propagated through the adjacent media. A portion of the energy generated at the surface is reflected back into the element. The net stress causing the element to deform is the sum of the forces resulting from the electrical energy across the element and the internally reflected mechanical energy. If the thickness of the piezoelectric element is one-half of the generated ultrasonic wavelength, these forces reinforce each other and the element vibrates at its resonant frequency [6]. A transducer is most efficient at transmitting and receiving energy when excited at its resonant frequency. Short pulses of ultrasound energy used in clinical echocardiography are not confined to a single frequency; generally a shorter pulse has a wider frequency range. A high-efficiency transducer is only sensitive to energy at its resonant frequency. To increase reception over a wider range of frequencies, piezoelectric elements are damped by the addition of absorbant backing material to transducers. They are also insulated from the transducer case to prevent ringing of the case, which may produce image artifact. Proper damping and insulation reduce transducer efficiency at a single frequency, but allow acceptable generation and reception of pulsed ultrasound energy with minimal artifact.

The propagation of an ultrasound wave away from the transducer can be analyzed using the principles of Huygen's construction. Ultrasound emanating from a point source is propagated in all three dimensions and therefore possesses a spherical wave front. The surface of a disc-shaped transducer may be considered to be an infinite number of separate elements, each radiating spherical waves away from the transducer as illustrated in figure 2-6. The separate waves are superimposed and reinforce themselves in such a way as to produce a beam with a planar wave front propagating in one direction. As the beam travels away from the transducer, it remains essentially parallel for a given distance and then begins to diverge. The parallel portion of the beam close to the transducer is called the near field; the divergent part is the far field, as shown in figure 2-7. The diagnostic power of ultrasound is best utilized when objects are examined within the near field because the beam is more parallel [7]. The range or length of the near field (l) is a function of the radius of the transducer (r) and the wavelength (λ) described by:

$$1 = r^2/\lambda$$

The near field may be lengthened by increasing the transducer radius or by decreasing the wavelength, which would require a higher ultra-

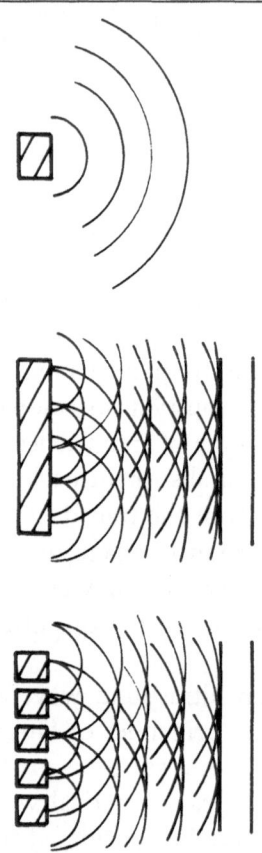

Figure 2-6. Wave fronts produced by single- and multiple-element transducers.

sound frequency. Larger transducers with higher frequencies also result in less divergence in the far field.

The beam width and divergence may be reduced by focusing the beam at a specific distance. This is done by using an acoustic lens on the surface of the transducer. Alternatively, focusing may be accomplished electronically using a transducer made up of many individual elements (see figure 2-8) [7]. Such a transducer is called a phased array transducer. By electronically timing the pulse wave of each element, a concave wave front is established with the resulting ultrasound beam focused at a specific depth. Electronic focusing enables changes to be made in focal zones by changing the firing times of the individual transducer elements; focusing occurs, however, only in one lateral dimension.

An ultrasound beam is a solid shape with three dimensions (figure

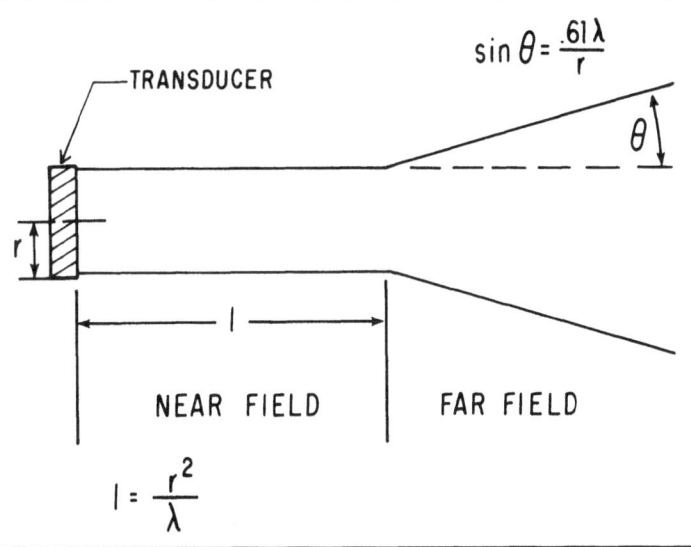

Figure 2-7. Nonfocused beam, divergent: l = length of near field, λ = wavelength, r = transducer radius, and θ = angle of divergence.

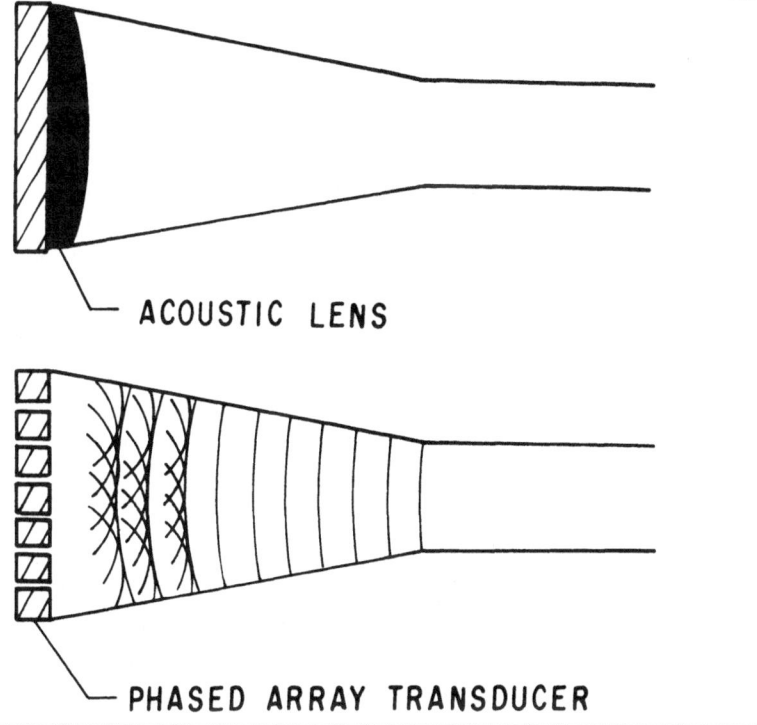

Figure 2-8. Focused ultrasound beams.

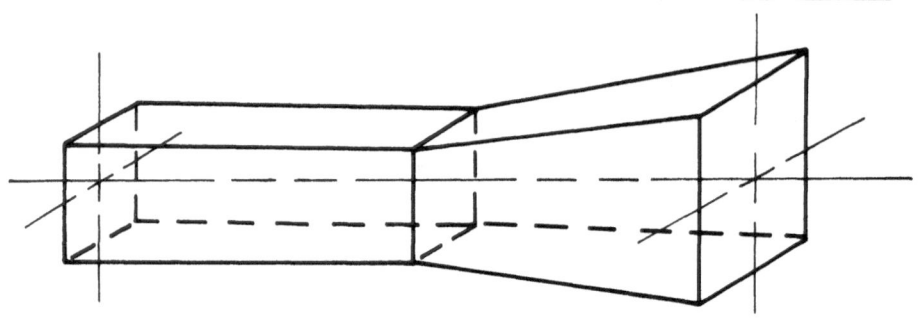

Figure 2-9. Three-dimensional shape of a rectangular ultrasound beam.

2-9). These include the axial dimension which is parallel to the direction of beam propagation and two lateral dimensions perpendicular to the beam, one vertical and one horizontal. A beam produced by a single circular transducer is cylindrical. A phased array transducer produces a beam with a rectangular cross section that is of greater intensity toward its center and lesser intensity near the lateral edges [7].

During an examination of the heart, the echocardiographer attempts to define and record an image of rapidly moving cardiac structures. The smallest distance between two discrete points that can be distinguished as separate defines the resolution of the system. Axial resolution refers to the ability to differentiate between two points lying along the axial dimension of the beam and lateral resolution refers to differentiation between two points lying side by side, perpendicular to the beam. Axial resolution is determined by the wavelength of the ultrasound and the duration of the transmitted pulse [6]. Shorter wavelengths (higher frequencies) and shorter pulse durations result in better axial resolution. Lateral resolution is determined by the beam width, with narrow beams having greater lateral resolution. Resolution is improved by selecting a transducer that produces short pulses of ultrasound with the highest frequency that allows adequate penetration, remembering that higher-frequency ultrasound is attenuated to a greater extent. The heart should be in the near field of a narrow beam or at the appropriate focal length in a focused beam. Amplification of the received signal is kept to a minimum so that only objects within the narrow high-intensity portion of the beam are recorded.

IMAGE DISPLAY: A, B, M AND 2D MODES

The instrument used to create and display an image with ultrasound is called an echograph. It must transmit electronic signals to the transducer which sends pulses of ultrasound to and receives echoes from the examined field. The reflected echoes are converted back into electrical voltages, amplified, and displayed in one of several formats for interpretation. By knowing the velocity of ultrasound, the time between transmission and reception of an ultrasound pulse is easily converted into the distance between the transducer and the reflecting structure. Distance is displayed in one dimension along one axis of a cathode-ray tube. The two classic formats for displaying echo images are the A mode and B mode (figure 2-10). The A mode displays objects as spikes on the oscilloscope with the height and width of the spike corresponding to the amplitude of the echo. The B mode displays echoes as dots, the brightness of which is proportional to the strength of the echo. The B mode format has supplanted A mode in clinical practice. An object that moves back and forth in the axial dimension will produce oscillation of the spike in A mode or dot in B mode. If time is displayed as a second dimension, while using B mode, the position of a reflecting structure is seen as a function of time. This format is called time motion or M-mode. An M-mode echogram of a structure oscillating in the axial direction would produce a sinusoidal curve. A limitation of M-mode echocardiography is that it only depicts structure and motion along a single dimensional axis as a function of time. An object that moves in a lateral direction is only periodically viewed as it passes in and out of the ultrasound beam; when it is viewed it always appears in the same position.

Within the last decade, it has become clinically feasible to produce two-dimensional images of the contracting heart with ultrasound. A two-dimensional image is formed by rapidly changing the axial direction of the ultrasound beam so that it passes through a sector of a plane that transects the heart. Figure 2-11 depicts a two-dimensional short-axis sector scan of the heart. Echoes from ultrasound pulses directed during one sweep through the sector are displayed in their corresponding positions on a cathode-ray tube to form a two-dimensional picture of the heart at that time. Repeated sweeps produce sequential pictures or frames during the cardiac cycle. If the frames are displayed at a sufficiently rapid rate, a television picture depicting a cross section of the dynamically contracting heart is produced.

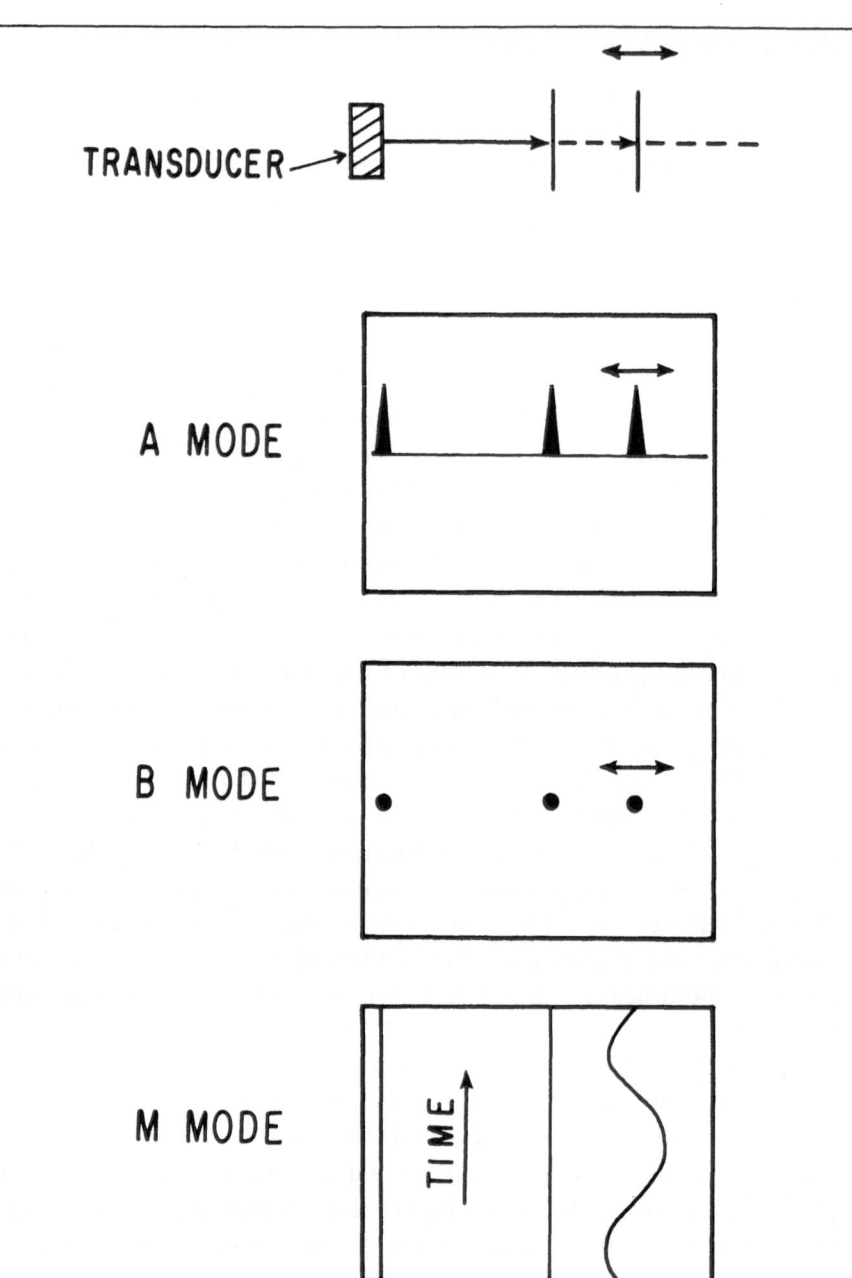

Figure 2-10. Image display modes.

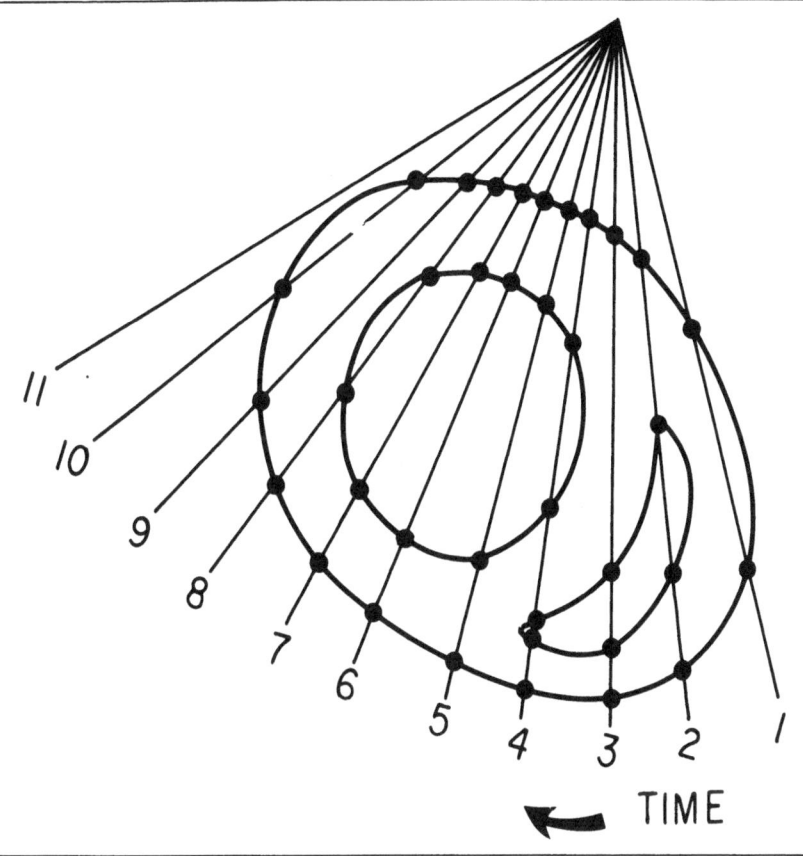

Figure 2-11. Sequence of ultrasound pulses during the sector sweep.

Although both mechanical and phased array transducer systems can be used to direct ultrasound pulses through the desired sector [8], phased array transducers are more commonly used in transesophageal two-dimensional echocardiography (figure 2-12). By varying the firing sequence of individual piezoelectric elements, wavelets are superimposed upon one another to produce a pulsed beam propagating in any desired direction. Each pulse is sequentially transmitted and received in a slightly different direction throughout a predetermined sector arc [9, 10].

The image quality obtained with two-dimensional echocardiography is limited by some physical constraints. A clear, continuously moving image requires a rapid frame rate with each frame including a large number of densely concentrated ultrasound echoes. As the frame rate increases, there is less time available for each frame, necessarily limiting the number of ultrasound echoes per frame. The maximum

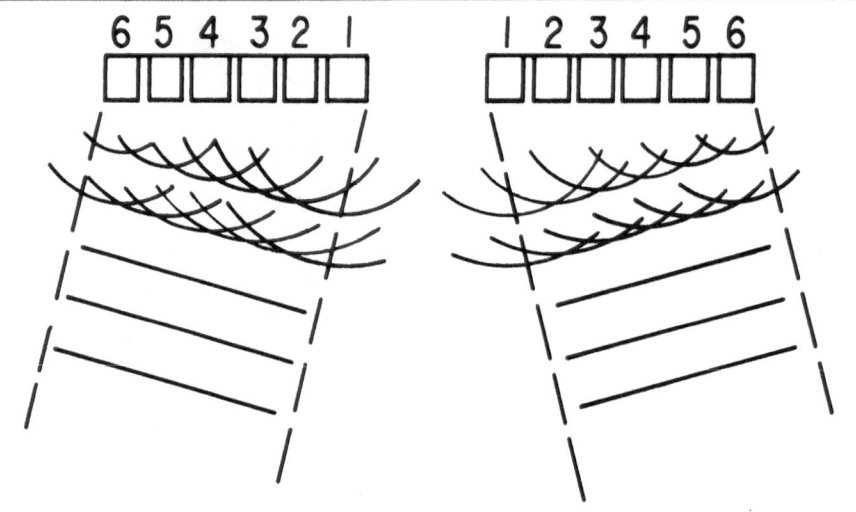

Figure 2-12. Phased array transducer directs ultrasound beam by varying sequence of pulses from individual elements.

rate of pulse transmission and reception, or pulse frequency, is limited by the velocity of ultrasound in human tissue ($1540 \, \mathrm{m \cdot s^{-1}}$) and the distance each pulse must travel, which is twice the depth of field to be examined. The line density, which is the number of ultrasound pulses per frame divided by the sector angle to be examined, therefore governs the quality of the image in a single stop-frame. An increase in depth of field or sector angle necessitates a decrease in line density for any given frame rate and results in poorer imaging.

FINER ADJUSTMENTS IN IMAGING: GRAY SCALE, GAIN CONTROLS

Several methods of electronic processing are used for the display of raw echo data to improve final image quality. As ultrasound echoes are received by the transducer, they are converted to voltages in the form of radio frequency signals. A radio frequency signal is processed to form a smooth wave encompassing its positive amplitude and is then electronically differentiated so that only the leading part of the signal is amplified. This tends to help separate echoes from closely spaced structures. A higher-intensity signal would be displayed in B mode by a brighter rather than a larger dot [7]. Transducers are capable of recording echoes varying in amplitude over a 100,000-fold range or 100 dB. Typical cathode-ray tubes are capable of displaying variations in brightness over only a 30-dB range. The amplitudes of transducer signals are electronically compressed, usually in a logarithmic fashion, to enable the cathode-ray tube to display echoes over the full dynamic range as areas of varying brightness or shades of gray. The term gray scale is used to describe the characteristic of displaying amplitude as a shade of gray, rather than an all-or-nothing format that appears only as black or white. Reject mechanisms are employed to eliminate recordings of weak echoes and low-amplitude noise. Variable gain is used to control the amplification of signals. Higher gain results in more echoes displayed in a brighter fashion, but decreases resolution and increases artifact. Because ultrasound is attenuated as it travels through tissue, echoes from far structures are deliberately enhanced and those from near structures are suppressed separately by time gain or depth compensation devices [7].

BIOLOGIC EFFECTS OF ULTRASOUND

A primary reason for the great interest in diagnostic echocardiography is the inherently small risk to the patient when compared with invasive procedures requiring catheterization or radiation exposure. Although thousands of patients have undergone diagnostic ultrasound procedures without reported complications, there is some reason for concern over the safety of exposure to high-intensity ultrasound. Early naval work with sonar demonstrated that small fish could be killed by high-intensity ultrasound [11].

Any potential biologic hazard is related to the total energy produced by a transducer and absorbed by the affected tissue. As discussed previously, the amount of energy produced per unit of time passing through a specific area is called intensity. The intensity of commercial transducers is measured in mW/cm^2 and the spatial average (SA) intensity is simply the power output divided by the surface area of the transducer. The actual intensity of an ultrasound beam is not uniform across its cross-sectional area but is greater toward the center of the beam; thus, the intensity at the center of the beam or spatial peak (SP) intensity is approximately three times the SA intensity. Evaluation of beam intensity of pulsed transducers used in M-mode or two-dimensional echocardiography is more complex. The "duty factor" is that fraction of time the probe is actually transmitting energy and is equal to the pulse duration multiplied by the pulse frequency. The temporal average (TA) power is the peak power during actual pulse production (temporal peak power) times the duty factor. The spatial average, temporal average intensity is the lowest of the various powers measured and is often quoted by manufacturers. However, the spatial peak temporal average (SPTA) intensity is probably a fairer assessment of the intensity to which tissue is subjected. Souquet and coworkers reported the SPTA intensity of their first transesophageal phased array probe to be $20 \, mW/cm^2$ [12]. No significant biologic effects have been found in tissues subjected to SPTA intensities less than $100 \, mW/cm^2$ [7].

Several investigations of the possible hazards of ultrasound have raised questions concerning genetic or teratogenic dangers. A critical review has concluded that, with the exception of extreme exposure conditions, evidence indicates that medical ultrasound diagnostic procedures are very unlikely to pose a genetic hazard [13]. This conclusion is supported by several more recent studies [14].

The local buildup of heat with possible thermal injury to the esophagus is of particular concern when using a transesophageal instrument. A transesophageal probe containing both horizontal and saggital arrays operated at $70 \, mW$ produced temperatures one degree above blood temperatures after extended use in cardiac surgical patients [15]. When operated at a maximum power of $140 \, mW$, temperature increases of 6–7 degrees were produced within 2 min. It is recommended that transducers be used at the minimum power necessary to provide adequate images. No esophageal burns have been reported in the literature.

Early investigations recommended diagnostic contrast radiologic examination of the esophagus prior to insertion of a transesophageal probe [16]. At the present time, there have been no reports of esophageal trauma from transesophageal echocardiography, even in patients who are fully heparinized for cardiopulmonary bypass. In patients without symptoms of esophageal disease, transesophageal echocardiography has thus far proven to be safe without prior radiographic examination.

Cucchiara, however, has reported a vocal cord injury in a patient who underwent a sitting craniotomy lasting several hours. It is possible that, with maximal neck flexion, the pressure exerted on the larynx by the endotracheal tube and the transesophageal probe resulted in vocal cord injury (personal communication).

REFERENCES

1. Halliday D, Resnick R: Fundamentals of physics. John Wiley and Sons, New York, 1974, pp 299–322.
2. Wells PNT: Absorption and dispersion of ultrasound in biological tissue. Ultrasound Med Biol 1:369–376, 1975.
3. Wells PNT: Ultrasonics in clinical diagnosis. Churchill Livingstone, New York, 1977, pp 3–17.

4. Carlson EN: Ultrasound physics for the physician: a brief review. J Clin Ultrasound 3:69–75, 1975.
5. Gregg EC, Palagallo GL: Acoustic impedance of tissue. Invest Radiol 4:357–363, 1969.
6. Wyman AE: Cross-sectional echocardiography. Lea and Febiger, Philadelphia, 1982.
7. Feigenbaum H: Echocardiography. Lea and Febiger, Philadelphia, 1980, pp 1–50.
8. Griffith JM, Henery WL: A sector scanner for real time two-dimensional echocardiography. Circulation 49:1147–1152, 1974.
9. Von Ramm OT, Thurstone FL: Cardiac imaging using a phased array ultrasound system. I. System design. Circulation 53:258–262, 1976.
10. Kisslo J, Von Ramm OT, Thurston FL: Cardiac imaging using a phased array ultrasound system. II. Clinical technique and application. Circulation 53:262–267, 1976.
11. Wood RW, Losmis AL: The physical and biological effects of high frequency sound waves of great intensity. Phil Mag 4:417–436, 1927.
12. Souquet J, Hanrath P, Zitelli L, Kremer P, Langenstein BA, Schluter M: Transesophageal phased array for imaging the heart. IEEE Trans Biomed Eng 29:707–712, 1982.
13. Thacker J: The possibility of genetic hazard from ultrasonic radiation. Curr Top Radiat Res Q 8:235–258, 1973.
14. Hill CR: Ultrasonics in clinical diagnosis. In: Wells PNT (ed). Churchill Livingstone, New York, 1977, pp 171–180.
15. Curling PF, Newsome LR, Rogers A, Hillard W, Sutherland J, Martin J, Nagle D, Waller JL: 2D-transesophageal echocardiography: a bidirectional phased array probe with temperature monitoring. Anesthesiology 61:A159, 1984.
16. Hanrath P, Schluter M, Langenstein BA, Polster J, Engel S: Transesophageal horizontal and saggital imaging of the heart with a phased array system: initial clinical results. In: Hanrath P, Bleifeld, W, Souquet J (eds) Cardiovascular diagnosis by ultrasound, transesophageal, computerized contrast, Doppler echocardiography. Martinus Nijhoff, The Hague, 1982, pp 280–288.

3. CARDIAC IMAGING FROM THE ESOPHAGUS; 2D ANATOMY; USE OF THE TRANSESOPHAGEAL PROBE

CARDIAC IMAGING FROM THE ESOPHAGUS

Effective use of transesophageal echocardiography requires some understanding of the transducer and the echograph, in addition to an appreciation of cardiac anatomy, as seen in cross section, from the esophagus. If the anatomy is understood, then the 2D image display can be understood, but the lack of established convention for transesophageal images results in some variation in the presentation and discussion of images in the literature. It becomes all the more important that users of transesophageal echocardiography define cardiac anatomy with standard cross-sectional views at specific levels. The correct identification of standard views, their use, and the essentials for displaying them are covered in this chapter.

THE TRANSDUCER

The transducer, measuring approximately 9 × 13 mm, is encased in the flexible shaft of a modified gastroscope from which the fiberoptics have been removed so that the whole assembly is smooth (figure 3-1). It can be angled in three planes by means of the two external controls and by rotating the scope manually about its long axis. A locking mechanism allows the operator to select an angle and maintain it

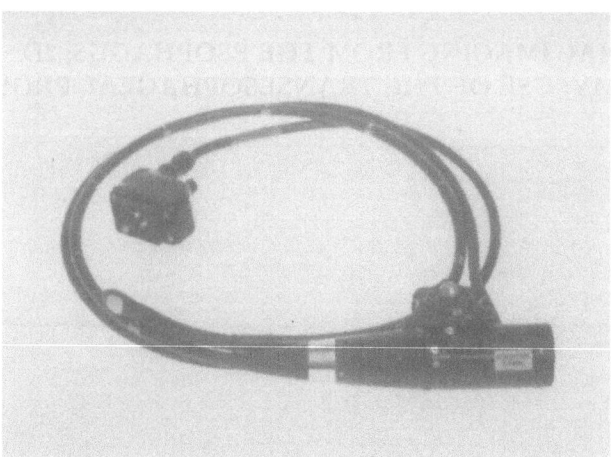

A

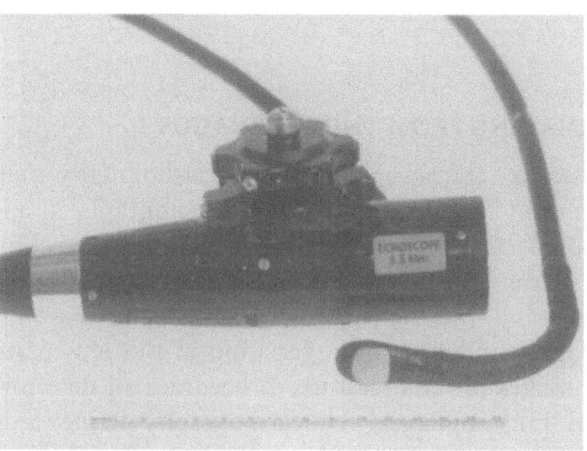

B

Figure 3-1. (A) Echoscope manufactured by the Diasonics Corporation. The shaft is marked every 10 cm to indicate the depth of insertion. (B) External controls for transducer angulation.

without holding continuous pressure on the controls. Most transesophageal views will be obtained by use of the flexion–extension control and rotation of the echoscope. Lateral angulation is seldom necessary (figure 3-2).

The ultrasound beam samples a thin, pie-shaped slice of tissue lying in a plane perpendicular to the long axis of the echoscope. Although manipulation of the transducer allows considerable flexibility, the

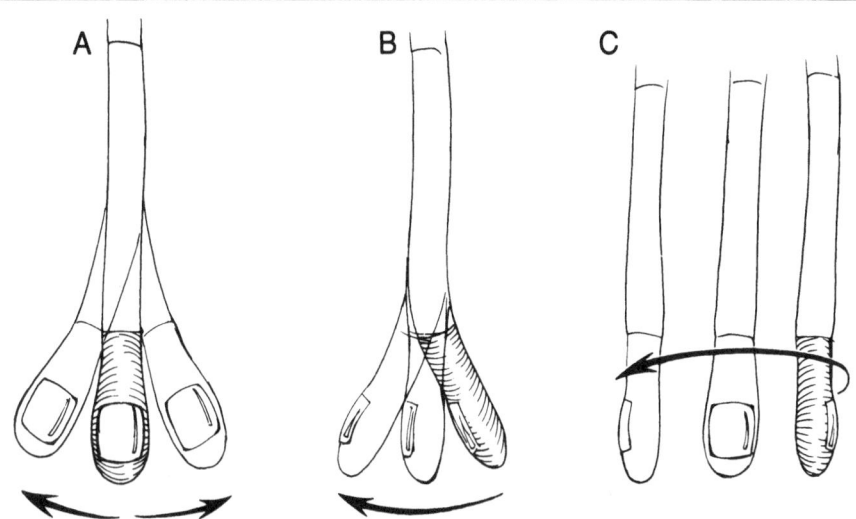

Figure 3-2. Range of transducer angulation: (A) lateral, (B) anterior–posterior flexion and extension, and (C) rotation.

constraints of the esophagus limit to some extent the ability to visualize cardiac structures.

ORIENTATION OF THE HEART WITHIN THE THORAX

Misconceptions regarding the normal orientation of the heart within the chest are common: illustrations sometimes depict the heart with its apex positioned inferiorly, and the ventricles lying side by side with the atria above. In fact, relative to the ventricles, the atria are situated posteriorly and only slightly superiorly. The cardiac apex is directed leftward, anteriorly, and somewhat inferiorly. Consequently, the interatrial and interventricular septa and the atrioventricular valves are oriented in the same direction. The right atrium becomes a right lateral chamber, and the left atrium a midline posterior chamber. The right ventricle is a right anterior chamber and the left ventricle is a left posterior chamber (figure 3-3). The diaphragmatic surface of the heart faces inferiorly except for its basal portion, which curves upward toward the atria. This basal, posteriorly facing part of the ventricles accounts for approximately one-third of the apex–base length.

RELATIONSHIP OF THE ESOPHAGUS TO THE HEART

The esophagus passes from the pharynx to the stomach with minor curvatures in the chest. In the superior mediastinum, it lies between

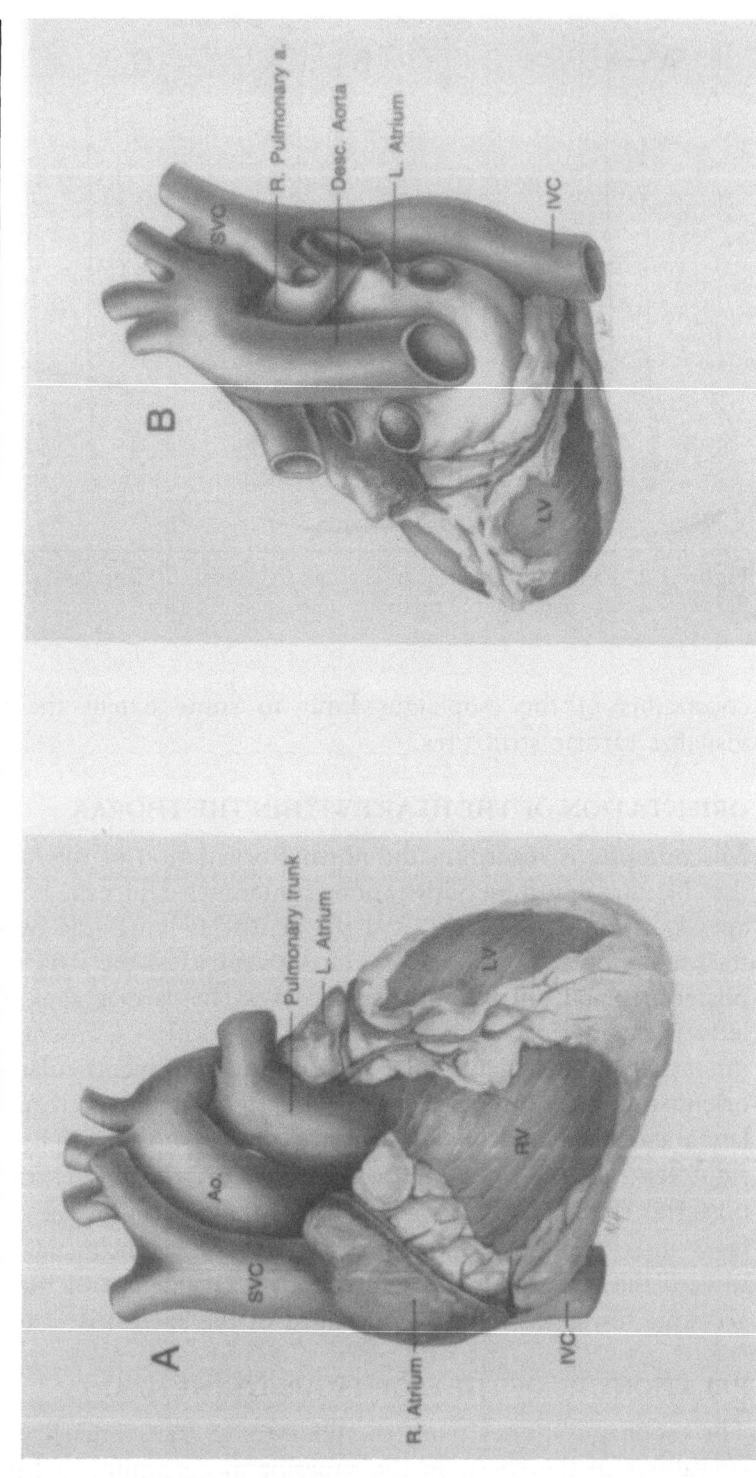

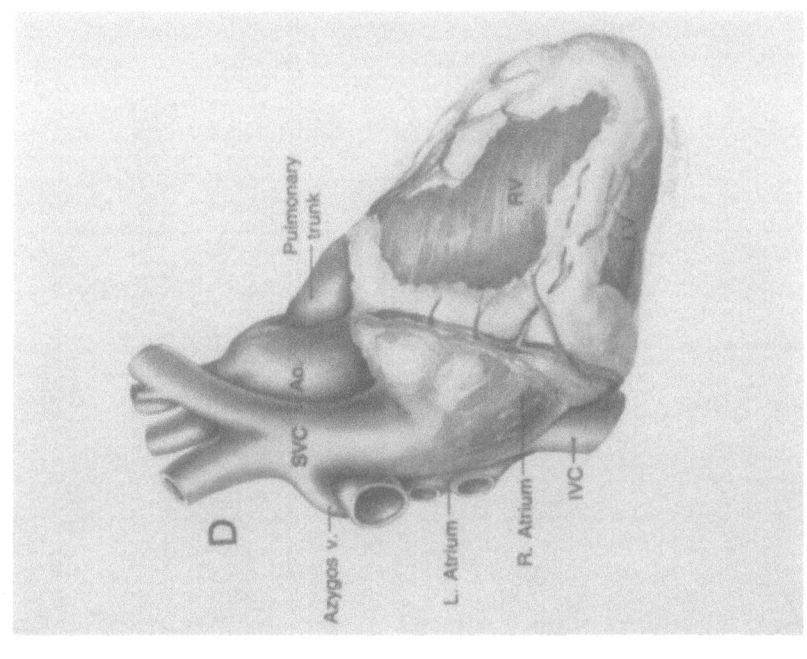

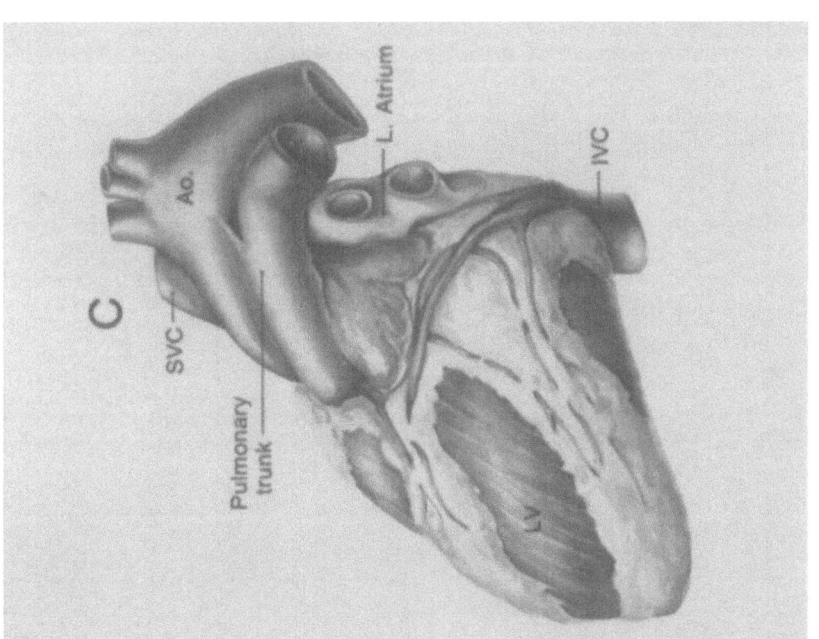

Figure 3-3. Orientation of the heart: (A) anterior, (B) posterior, (C) left lateral, and (D) right lateral.

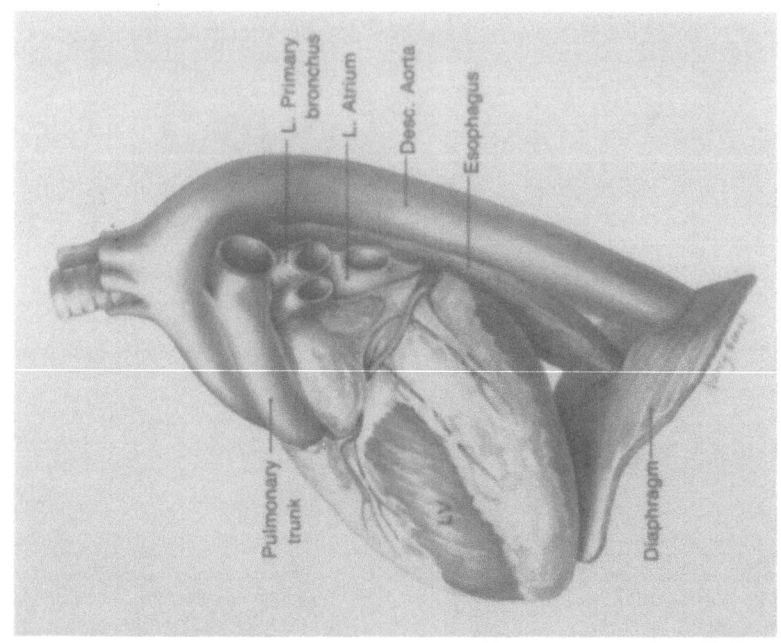

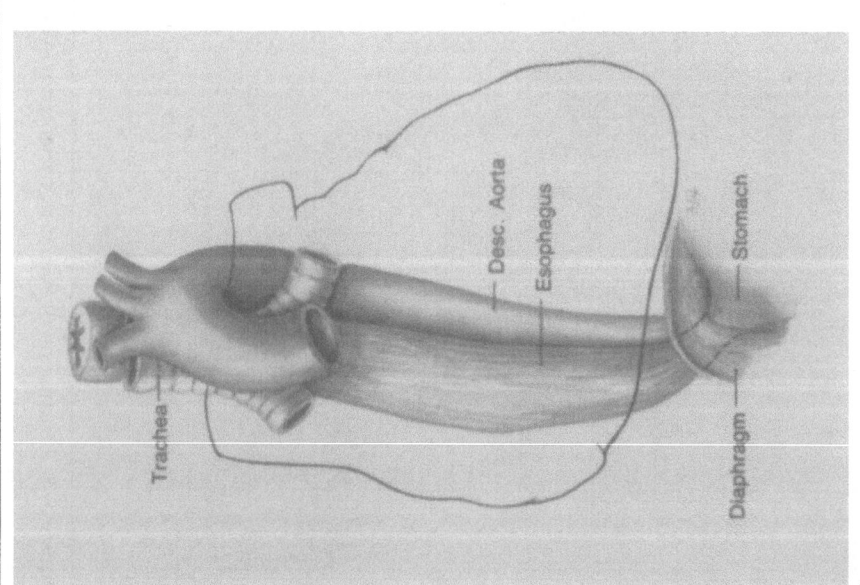

Figure 3–4. Position of the esophagus relative to the heart: (A) anterior view and (B) lateral view.

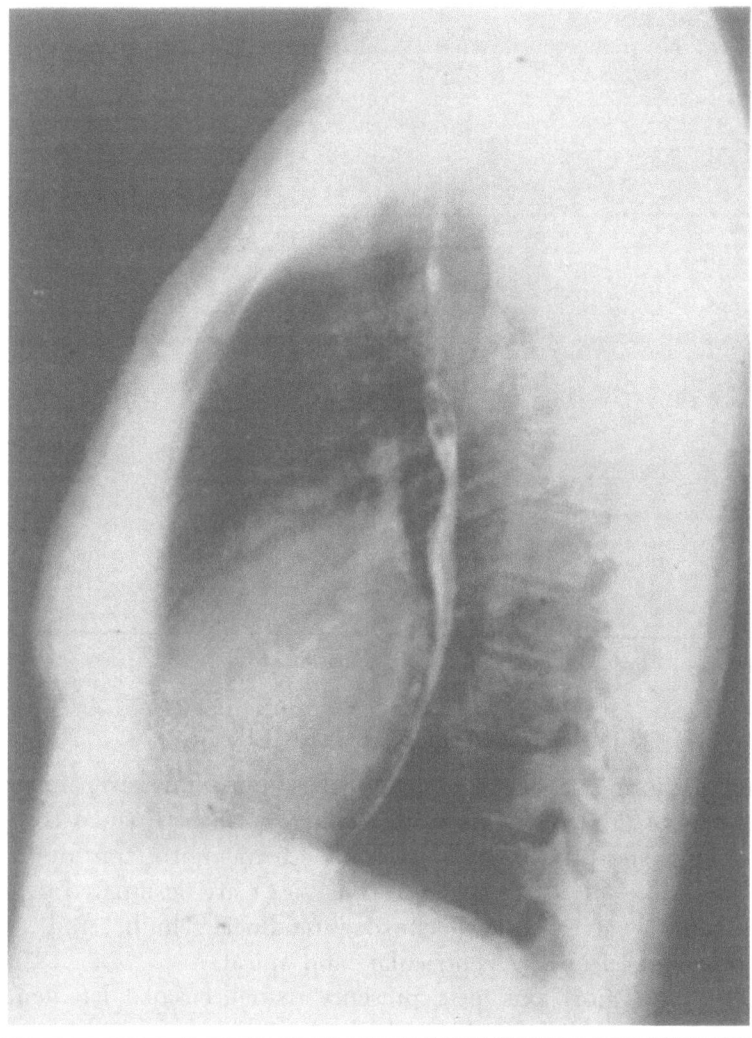

Figure 3-5. Barium swallow radiograph in an erect patient. In the supine patient the heart falls more posteriorly.

the trachea and the vertebral column slightly to the left of the median plane. It then descends behind and to the right of the aortic arch to lie in the posterior mediastinum on the right side of the descending aorta. It passes in front of the lower thoracic aorta and leftward, before passing through the diaphragm into the stomach (figure 3-4A and B). The heart lies immediately anterior to the esophagus, so that the ultrasound transducer is separated from the left atrium and left ventricle only by the esophageal wall (figure 3-5).

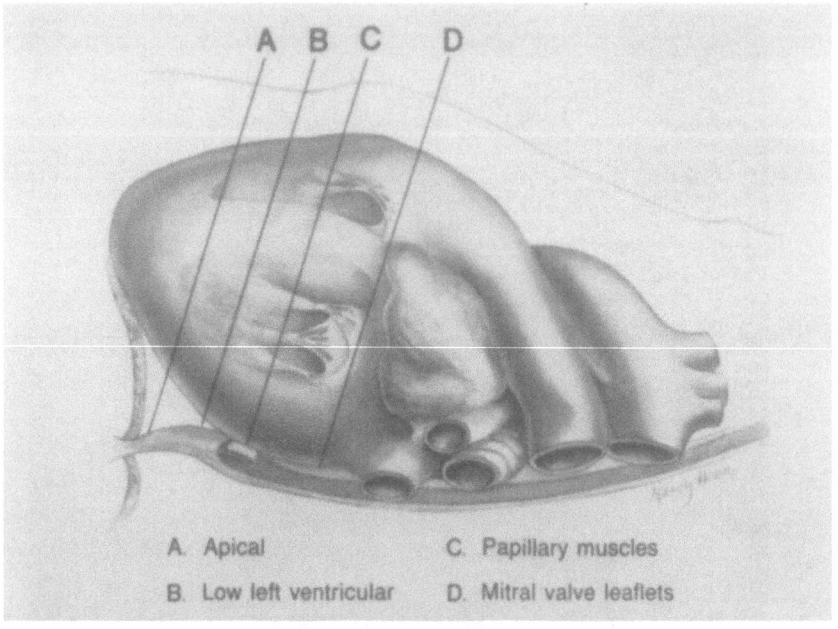

Figure 3-6. Short-axis levels of the left ventricle.

SHORT-AXIS IMAGING OF THE VENTRICLES

When the long axis of the esophagus lies approximately parallel to the long axis of the left ventricle, the ventricle can be imaged completely in multiple short-axis views by simply advancing the transducer down the esophagus (figure 3-6). Short-axis views are designated by a level, i.e., mitral valve leaflets, chordae tendineae, high, mid, or low papillary muscles, low ventricular, and apical.

The apical short-axis view presents a small circular left ventricular (LV) cavity contained within a thick symmetric ventricular wall. This apical view is defined as the lowest view of the left ventricle with a clearly discernible cavity area. Just proximal to the apical view, a low LV level may be defined below the level at which the papillary muscles indent the LV cavity. Here also the cavity and the ventricular wall appear circular and symmetric, though the cavity area is larger than at the apical level (figure 3-7). As the cross-sectional short axis is taken more proximally, the papillary muscles begin to appear, indenting the ventricular cavity. They represent important anatomic landmarks for the echocardiographer. In longitudinal cross section, it can be seen that the papillary muscles extend for about one-third of the LV cavity length (figure 3-8). There are two papillary muscle bodies,

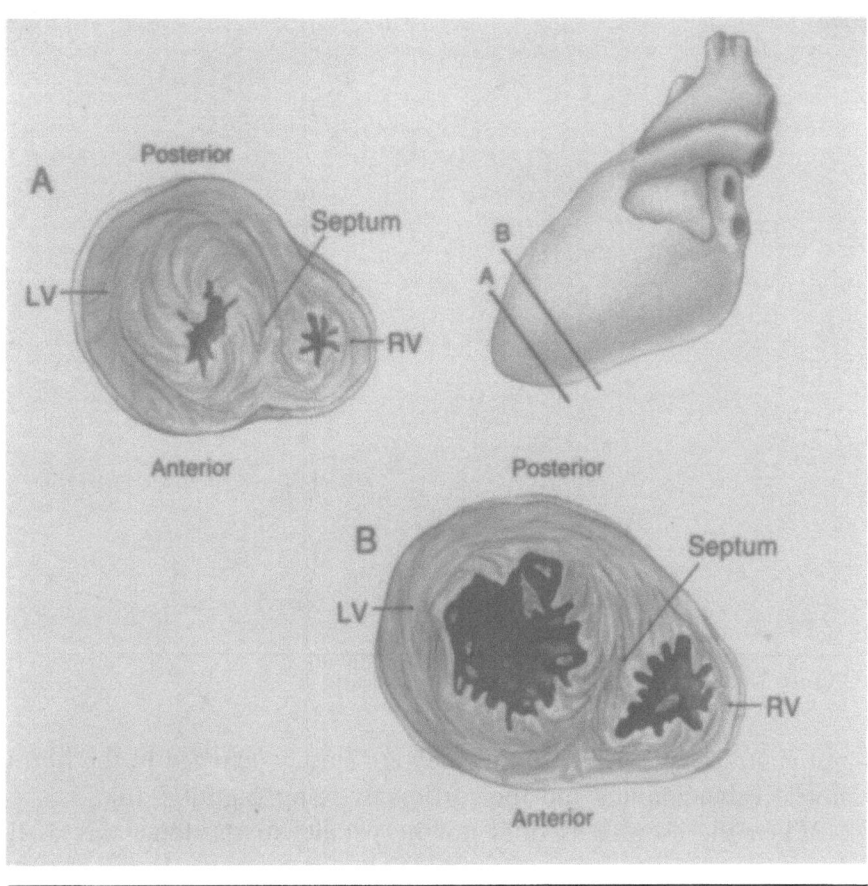

Figure 3-7. Left and right ventricles in cross section: (A) apical level and (B) low ventricular level.

anterior and posterior, which arise from the ventricular wall as single trunks and divide variably into two or more trunks before joining the chordae tendineae. Three papillary muscle levels are sometimes described (figure 3-9): the low papillary muscle level lies at the level where the muscles first appear, indenting the ventricular cavity: the midpapillary level is that at which the two muscle trunks appear as well-defined structures, contiguous with the ventricular wall; the high-papillary level is that at which the muscles appear as discrete bodies, separate from the ventricular wall. Immediately above the papillary muscles, the chordae tendineae appear, and the mitral valve leaflets. The latter exhibit a characteristic fish-mouth appearance in a short-axis cross section. At this level, the LV cavity appears circular. However, the ventricular walls may not appear symmetric and may

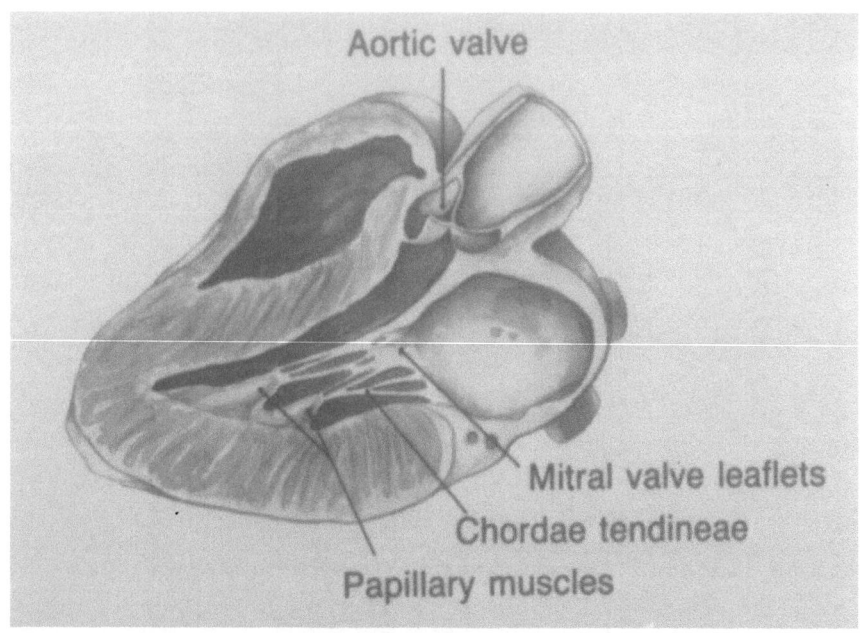

Figure 3-8. Longitudinal section through the heart.

not contract symmetrically, as they are closely attached to the fibrous mitral valve annulus and the aortic valve ring (figure 3-10).

When the esophagus does not lie parallel to the long axis of the heart, the identification of multiple short-axis views becomes more difficult. In short obese persons, imaging is frequently unsatisfactory for this reason, as the esophagus becomes displaced from the heart by a high diaphragm. The orientation of the ultrasound beam perpendicular to the long axis of the esophagus lends itself to short-axis imaging rather than long-axis imaging, but this is generally quite satisfactory for the purposes of intraoperative monitoring. It is desirable that the transesophageal echocardiographer obtain true short-axis views, representing cross-sectional planes at right angles to the long axis of the heart. True short-axis views are identified by the appearance of a circular ventricular cavity rather than an elliptical, oblique section, which indicates that transducer angulation is incorrect (figure 3-11).

IMAGING THE LONG AXIS OF THE HEART AND SUPRAVENTRICULAR STRUCTURES

With a transesophageal transducer, the best approximation to a long-axis view of the heart is obtained by moving the transducer up behind

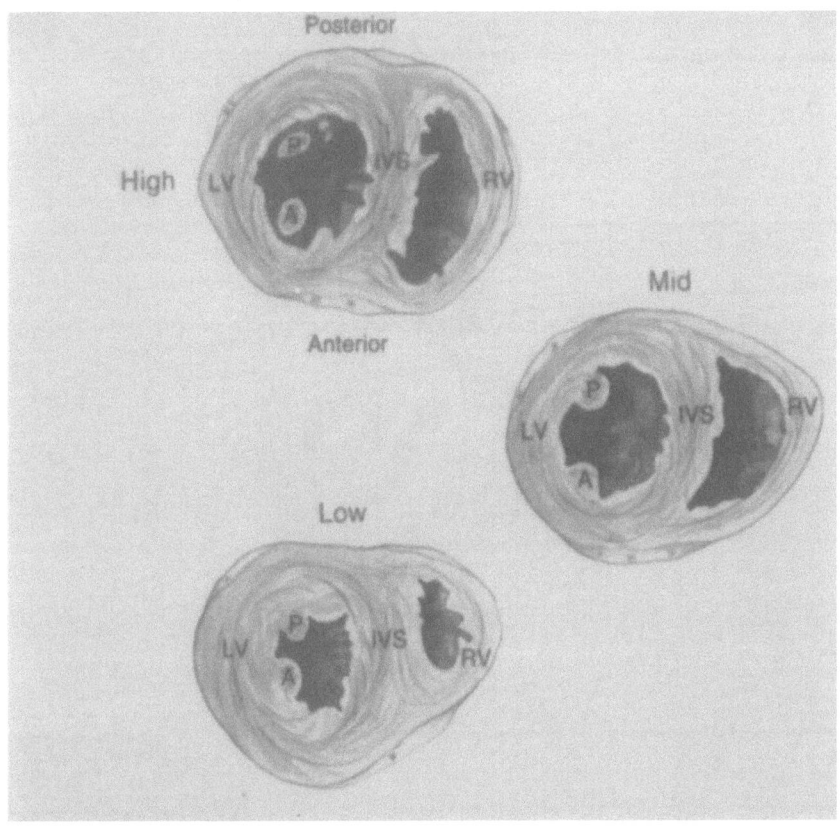

Figure 3-9. Short-axis views at three papillary muscle levels: LV = left ventricular free wall, RV = right ventricular free wall, IVS = intraventricular septum, P = posterior papillary muscle, and A = anterior papillary muscle.

the left atrium and angling the beam downward toward the cardiac apex. Invariably this foreshortens the heart somewhat, because the beam cannot be directed precisely through the apex (figure 3-12).

From a similar position behind the left atrium, the ultrasound beam can be directed anteriorly to image the ventricular outflow tracts and the great vessels (figure 3-13).

IMAGE NOMENCLATURE AND DISPLAY

Formal image nomenclature has not been designated for transesophageal views; however, the standards prescribed by the American Society of Echocardiography for transthoracic views can to a large extent be adapted for transesophageal imaging [1].

What is less well standardized is the image display. The ultrasound

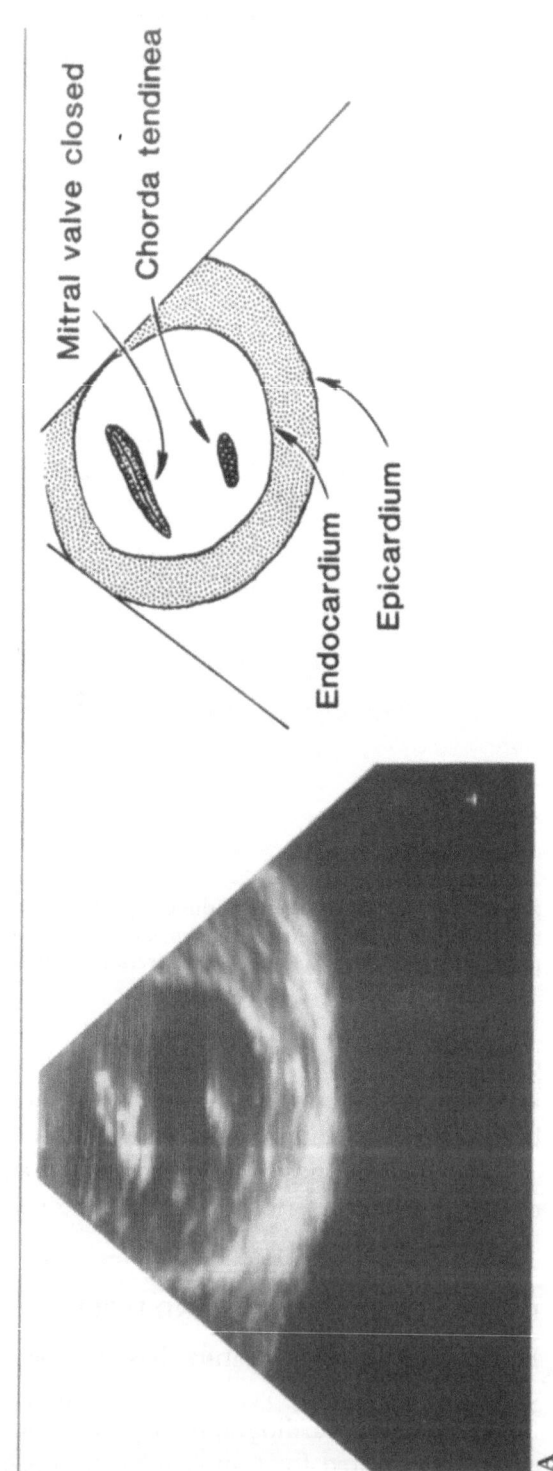

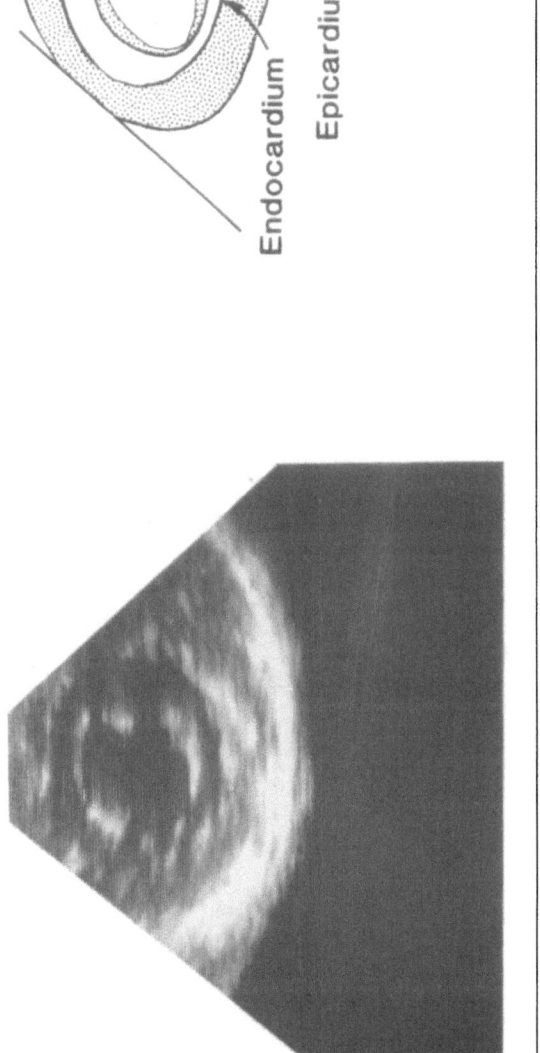

Figure 3-10. Short-axis image at the mitral valve level: (A) mitral valve leaflets closed in systole and (B) mitral valve leaflets open in diastole.

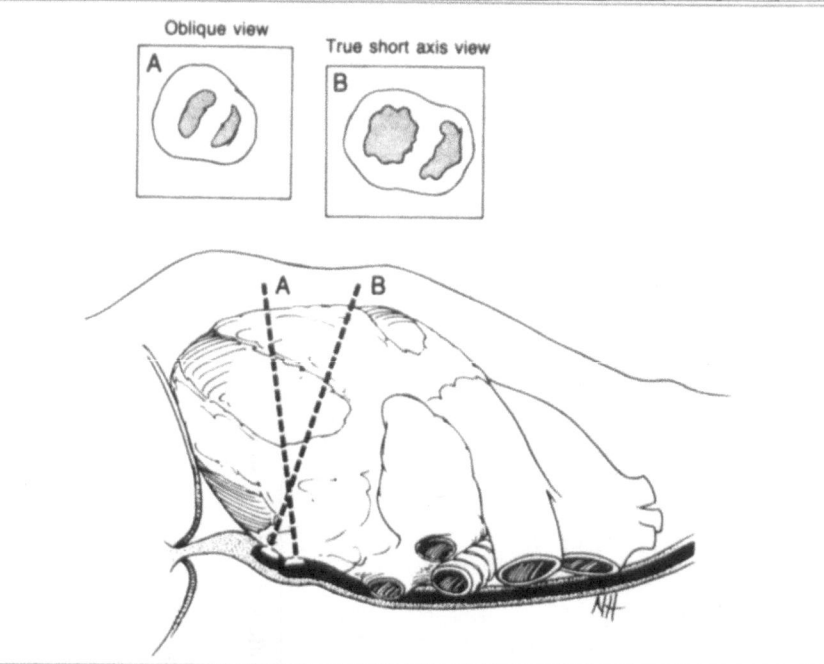

Figure 3-11. Transducer angulation for short-axis views: (A) incorrectly angled transducer and (B) correctly angled transducer.

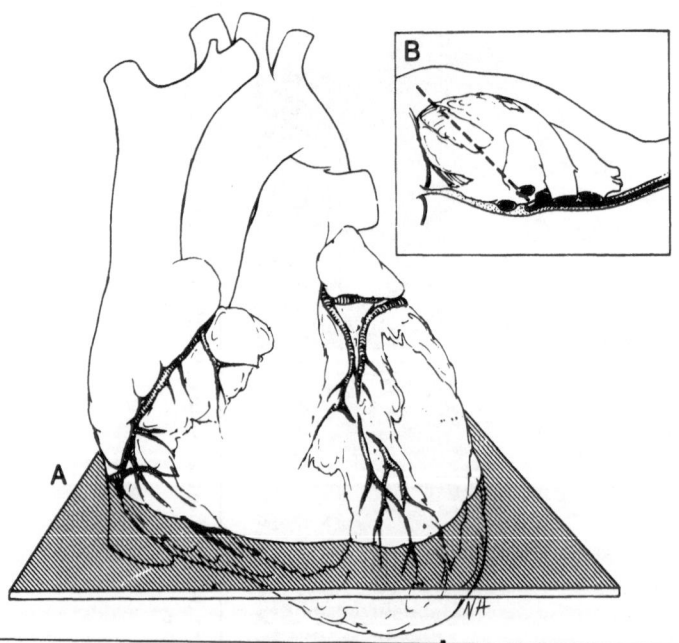

Figure 3-12. Long-axis imaging: (A) plane of image and (B) position of echoscope in the supine position.

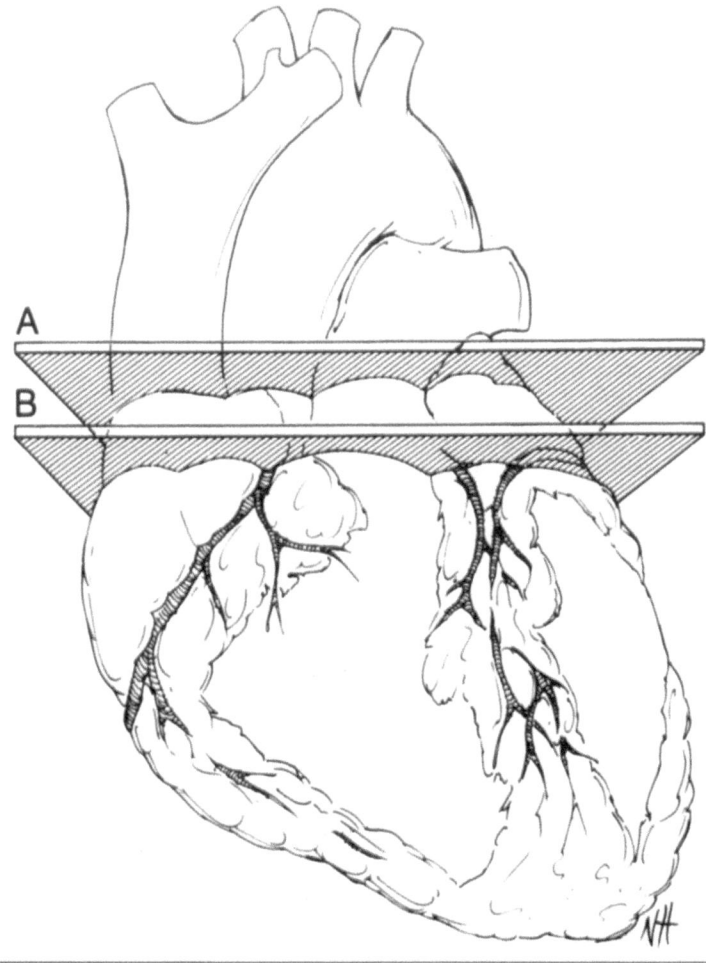

Figure 3-13. Imaging plane for supraventricular structures: (A) great vessels and atria and (B) ventricular outflow tracts, aortic valve and atria. The anteriorly placed pulmonary valve is not well seen with transesophageal images.

transducer can be represented on the videoscreen image at the top of the screen with the left ventricle, in a short-axis view, appearing immediately adjacent, and the right ventricle appearing off to the right side (figure 3-14A).

An inversion switch allows the operator to invert the image so that the transducer appears at the bottom of the image, but with left right orientation as before (figure 3-14B).

Alternatively, some echographs permit left–right inversions, such that the operator visualizes cardiac structures from an opposite perspective (figure 3-14C).

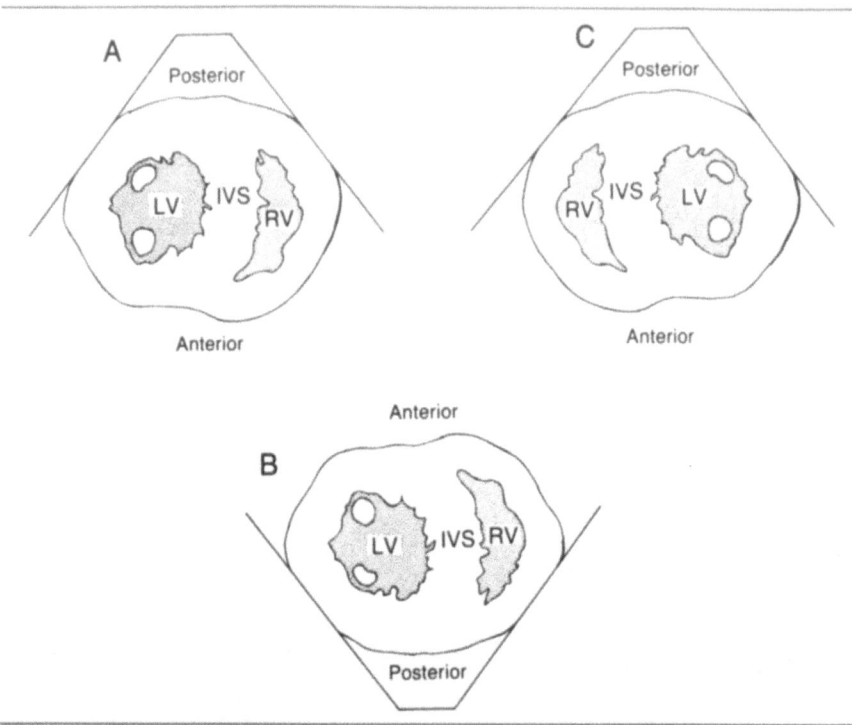

Figure 3-14. Alternative image orientations (short axis).

Illustrations in this book are oriented as shown in figure 3-14A. The long-axis view then appears in a transesophageal image as shown in figure 3-15, with the left atrium closest to the transducer and the left ventricle appearing on the left side of the image.

For descriptive purposes, the American Society of Echocardiography recommends that the ventricular walls be divided into three regions along the long axis of the heart. For this four-chamber view, a reference line is constructed through the mitral and tricuspid annuli. The ventricles are divided by parallel lines to establish the basal, mid, and apical regions. The basal portion extends from the valve annuli to the tips of the papillary muscles, the mid portion from the tips to the bases of the papillary muscles, and the apical region includes the remainder of the ventricle. The ventricular free walls are considered to extend from the cardiac apex to the atrioventricular valve annuli, and are bounded anteriorly and posteriorly by their attachments to the interventricular septum. Although the septum constitutes a part of both the right and left ventricles, its thickness and spatial configuration suggest that it is an anatomic and functional part of the left

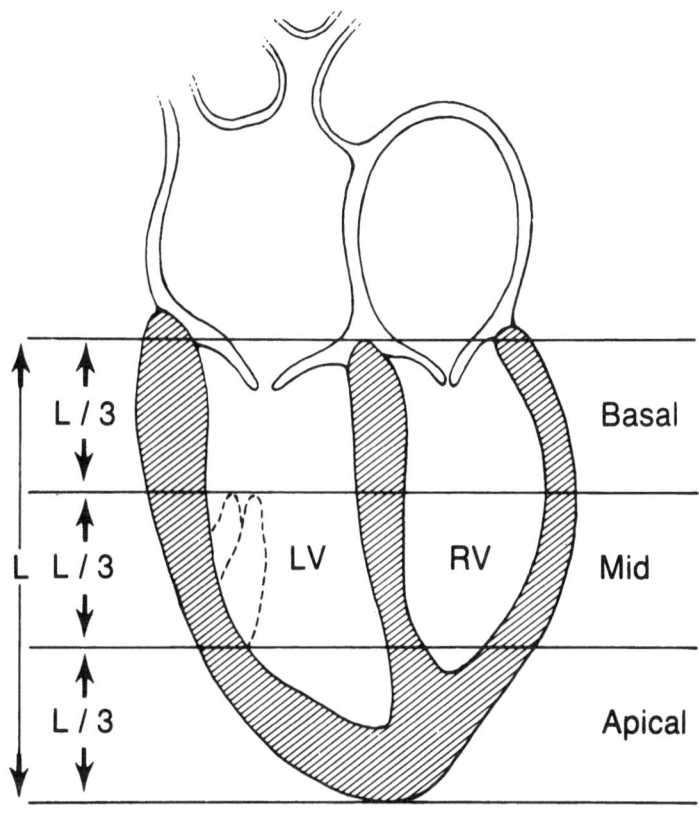

Figure 3-15. Diagram of the long-axis image.

ventricle. In cross section, the septum forms approximately 40% of the LV wall, contributing to the circular LV cavity appearance; the right ventricle appears crescentic, and thin walled, relative to the left ventricle.

Figure 3-16 illustrates the recommended segmental divisions of the short-axis view, with the left ventricle being divided into eight segments. The orientation of the segments is initiated by a 0–180° line bisecting the ventricular cavity parallel to a line drawn between the medial and lateral commissures of the mitral valve, or at a papillary muscle level, by a line drawn through the center of the papillary muscles. From this reference line, a second orthogonal line is placed at 90° and the quandrants so produced are further bisected to create octants. Since the apical region has a much smaller cross-sectional area, this region is divided into four segments only. Extension of the septal divisions into the right ventricle creates three segments of the

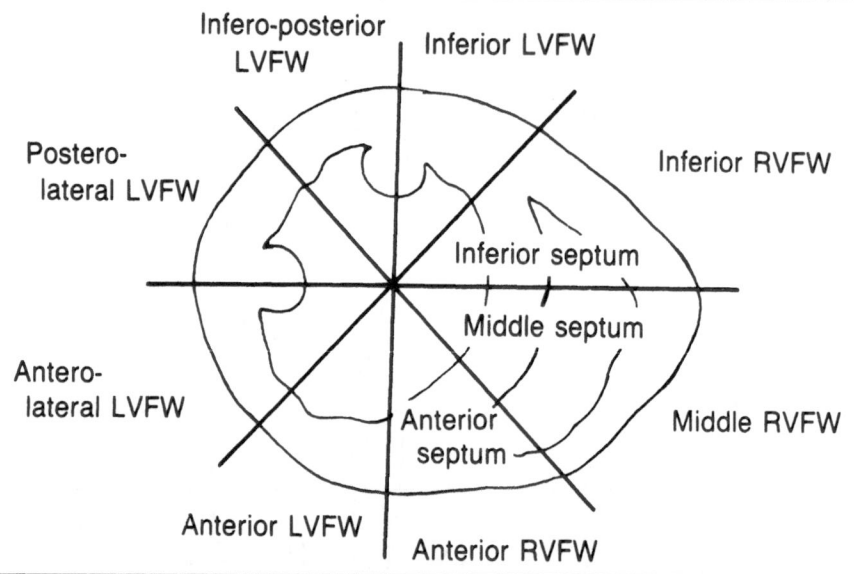

Figure 3-16. Midventricular short axis view. LVFW = left ventricular free wall, and RVFW = right ventricular free wall.

right ventricular free wall. The use of this standard nomenclature allows comparison of ventricular images produced with contrast ventriculography or radionuclide angiography. In relating regional wall motion to coronary perfusion, however, many investigators have employed a simpler system of segmental division, which is more practical for everyday use. Thus, the short-axis views at basal or midventricular levels can be divided into four segments only: posterior or inferior, lateral, anterior, and septal. The apex is considered as one segment.

TECHNICAL ASPECTS OF TRANSESOPHAGEAL IMAGING

Whether awake or anesthetized, patients may be imaged in the supine position. It has generally been recommended that awake patients be held fasting for 4–8 h prior to transesophageal imaging. Introduction of the scope in awake patients may be accompanied by slight gagging, as with routine flexible gastroscopy. This is overcome by topical anesthesia to the pharynx with tetracaine or lidocaine, and 5–10 mg of intravenous diazepam. For anesthetized patients whose airway is protected by an endotracheal tube, no such preparation is necessary. A prior history of dysphagia, upper gastrointestinal bleeding or history of esophageal varices, or any bleeding diathesis should be reason to consider carefully the indications for transesophageal echocardio-graphy. A barium swallow may sometimes be indicated to define esophageal anatomy. In the absence of any history suggesting esophageal pathology, however, it has not been the authors' practice to obtain routinely a barium swallow. Transesophageal echocardio-graphy has also been extensively used in patients who are fully heparinized for cardiopulmonary bypass without any reports of esophageal bleeding.

Prior to use, the echoscope should be inspected for cracks and signs of wear. The controls should be released from the locked position so that the echoscope can slide freely through the pharynx and lub-ricating gel should be applied generously before use. The echoscope can usually be introduced blindly into the esophagus; occasionally it will be useful to do it under direct vision with a laryngoscope. No resistance should be encountered as the transducer is advanced to 40 or 50 cm from the incisors. As the echoscope is gradually withdrawn from this position, a beating structure will come into view (figure 3-17). Often without any use of the controls, a good short-axis image will be produced, but if the long axis of the heart is displaced away from the esophagus some anterior angulation of the transducer may be necessary to bring the left ventricle into view. Obese patients in the supine position sometimes present this problem as the abdominal contents push the diaphragm cephalad and cause the heart to lie in a more transverse position. It is possible to image the heart from the stomach, provided that the transducer can be angled ventrally enough to lie in contact with the gastric wall. In this way, short-axis images may be obtained in some patients. In general, we obtain short-axis images from the esophagus.

After examining the left ventricle in short-axis views from the apex to the level of the mitral valve, the echoscope can be further with-drawn until it lies behind the left atrium. At this level, an oblique sectional view through the mitral valve and aortic outflow tract often appears (figure 3-18). The aortic valve leaflets appear as three lines, open in systole and closed in diastole.

Angulation of the transducer inferiorly at this level brings the four-chamber long-axis view on the videoscreen, allowing examination of the mitral and tricuspid valves. The anterior mitral valve leaflet lies adjacent to the interventricular septum and the posterior leaflet is more lateral in this view (figure 3-19).

Releasing the transducer angle, the echoscope can be withdrawn another centimeter to image a plane through the aortic valve. The

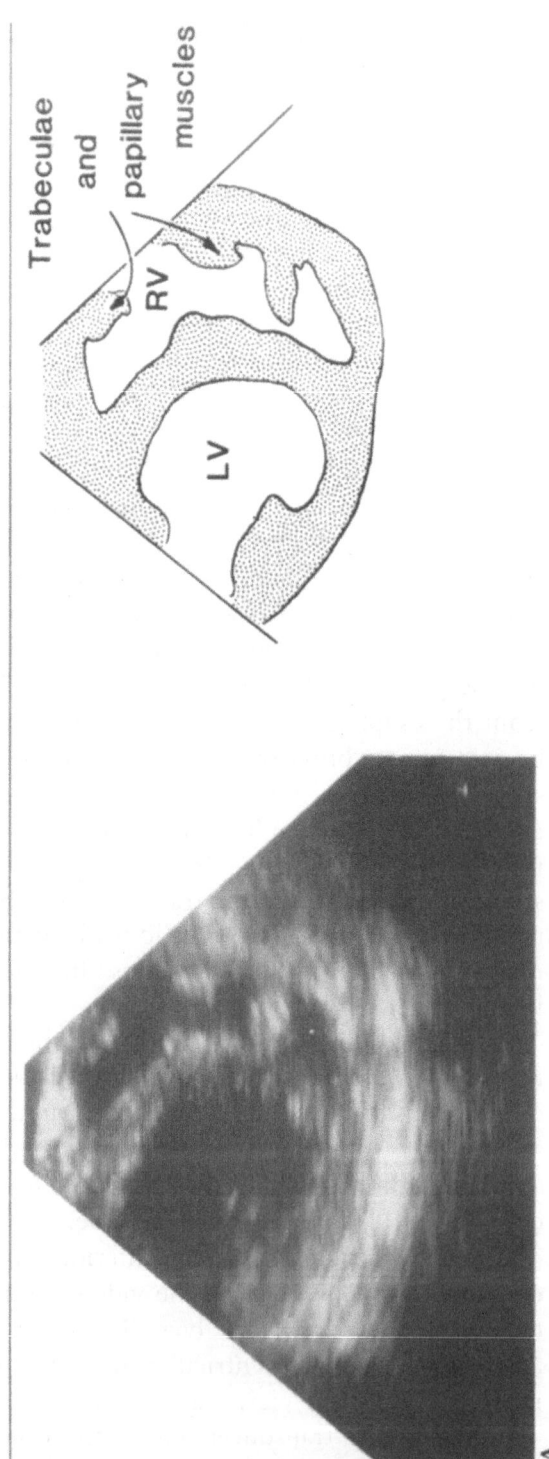

Trabeculae and papillary muscles

RV

LV

A

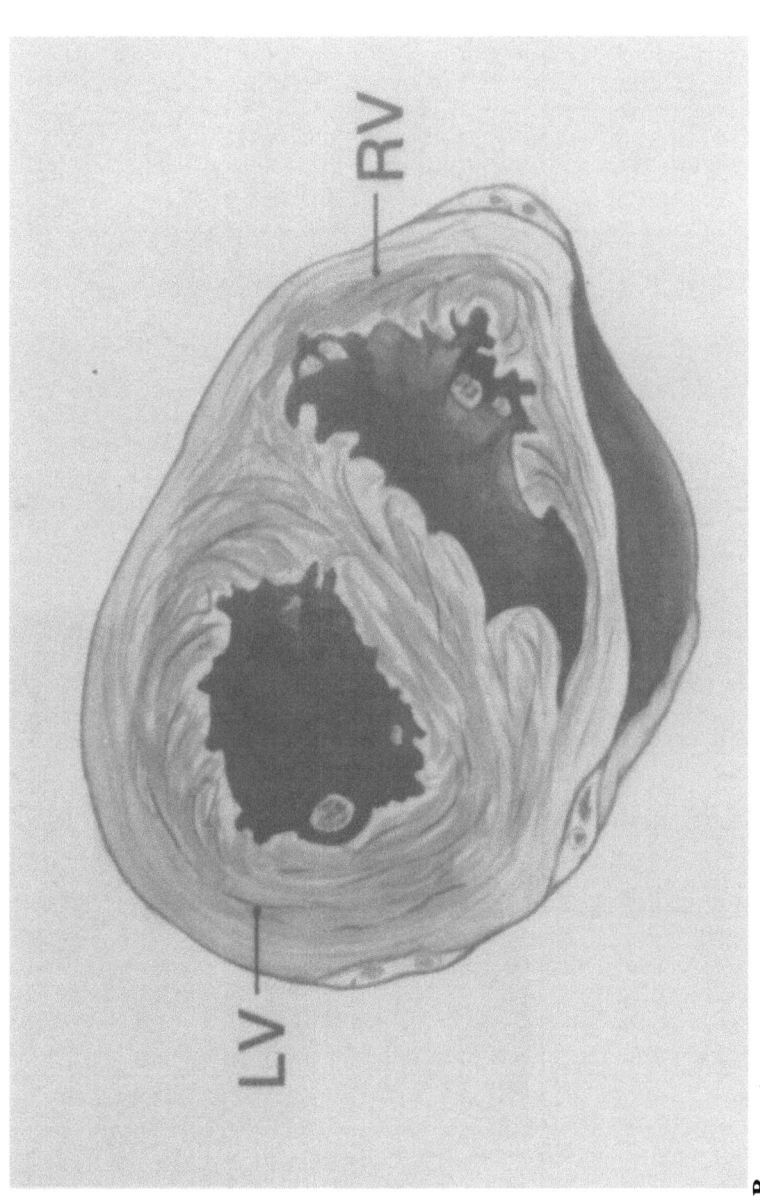

B

Figure 3-17. (A) short-axis two-chamber image: LV = left ventricle, and RV = right ventricle. (B) Drawing of corresponding anatomic section.

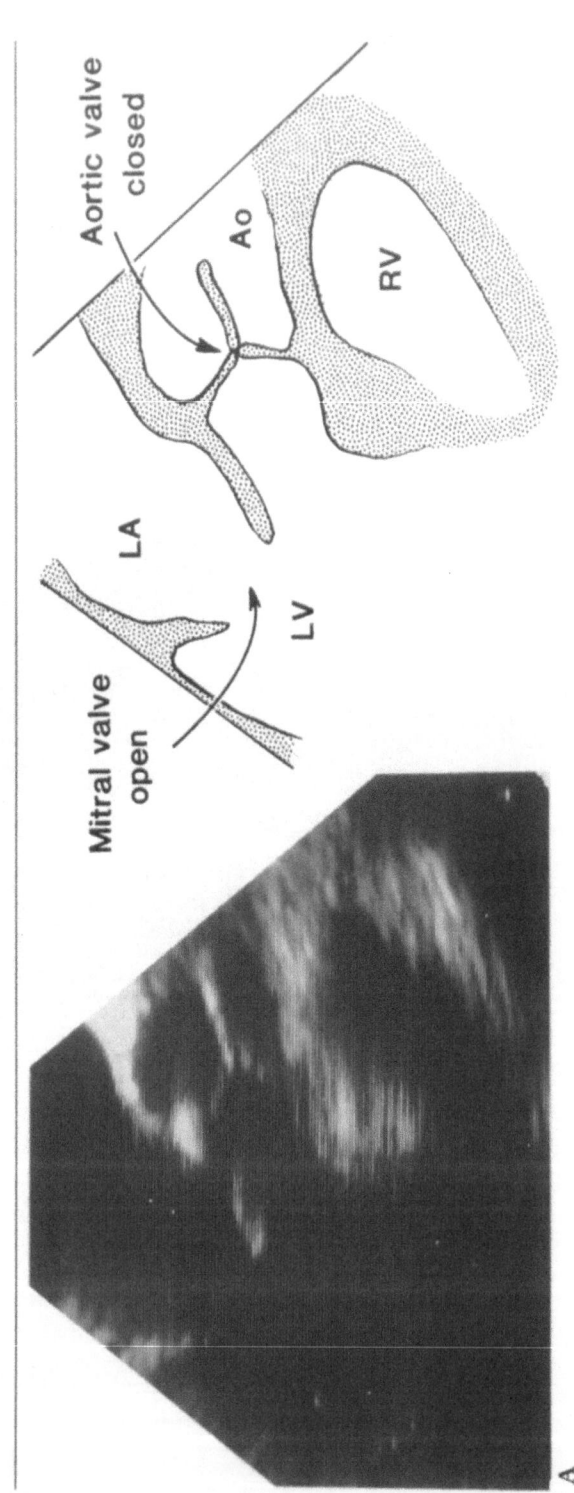

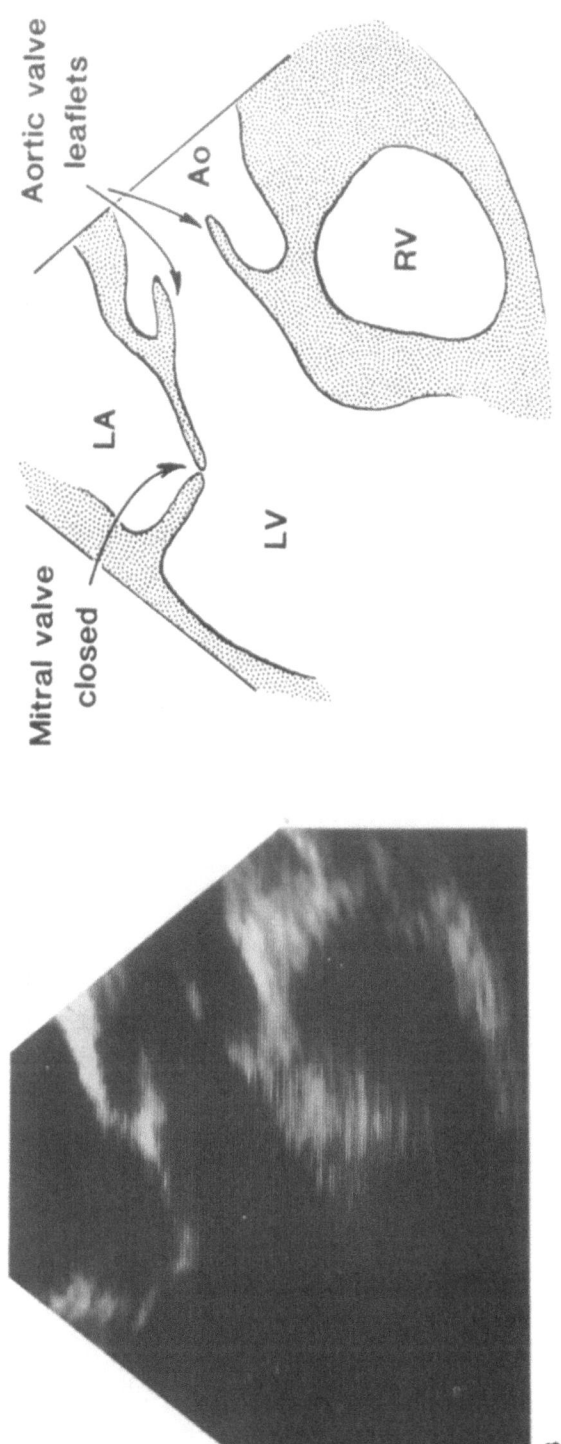

Figure 3-18. Oblique sectional image: (A) diastole and (B) systole. RV = right ventricle, LV = left ventricle, LA = left atrium, and AO = aorta.

52

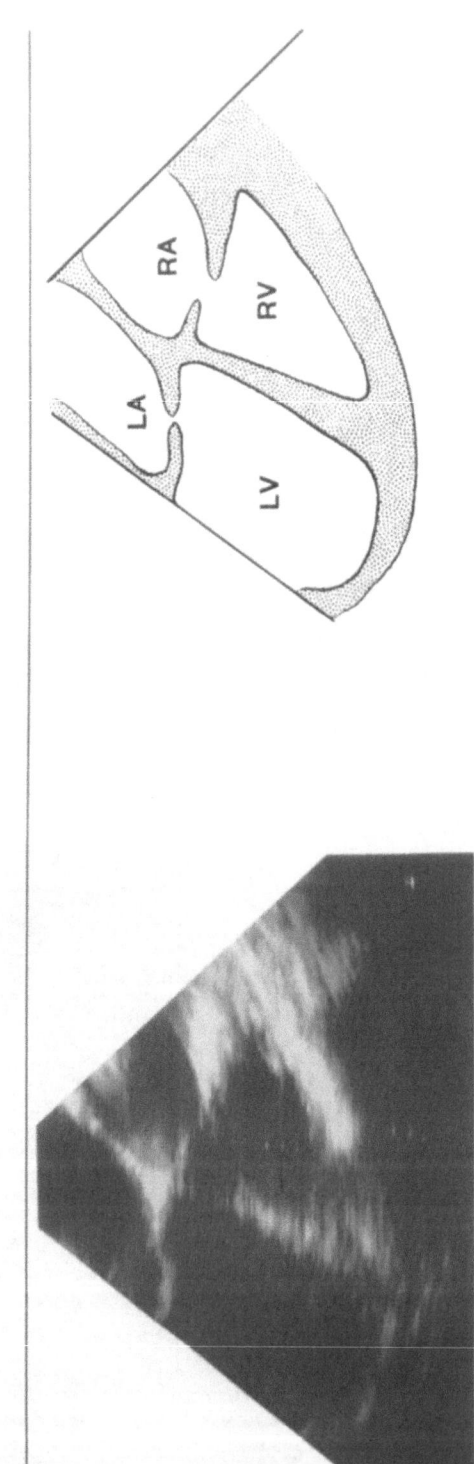

Figure 3-19. Four-chamber long-axis view: RV = right ventricle, LV = left ventricle, RA = right atrium, and LA = left atrium.

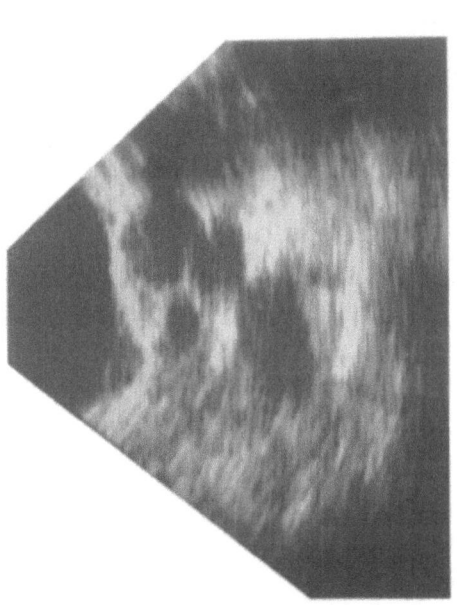

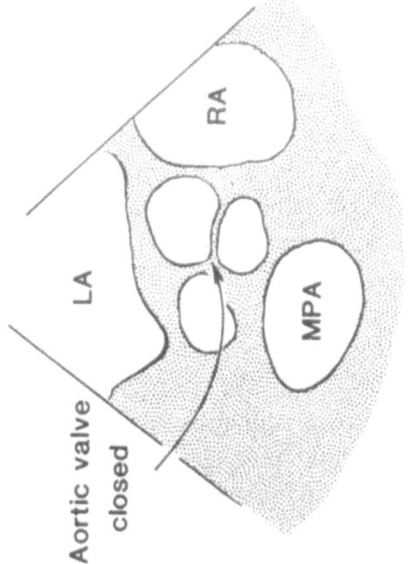

Figure 3–20. Aortic valve cross-sectional image: LA = left atrium, RA = right atrium, and MPA = main pulmonary artery.

three valve leaflets can be identified and the aorta appears circular in cross section. Slight withdrawal of the echoscope from this position brings the sinuses of Valsalva into view (figure 3-20) and then more cephalad the aorta becomes elliptical in cross section as it arches laterally and posteriorly. Above this level, imaging is lost as the ultrasound beam encounters air in the tracheobronchial tree. From the position behind the left atrium suitable for imaging the aortic valve, slight clockwise rotation of the transducer brings the interatrial septum into view. Atrial septal defects can be examined and contrast injection used to demonstrate interatrial shunting.

For intraoperative monitoring of global and regional LV function, the echoscope will be left in a stable position for continuous observation. After a general echocardiographic examination of the heart as described above, the echoscope is generally returned to the postion that provides a short-axis view at a midpapillary muscle level. In awake patients, a diagnostic examination should take about 10 min.

The actual time taken will depend largely on the skill of the operator with the topical anesthesia and manipulation of the transducer. Otherwise there are a limited number of views possible within the confines of the esophagus. Whereas this has its disadvantages, it also makes the technique easier to learn than transthoracic echocardiography.

REFERENCES

1. Henry WL, DeMaria A, Feigenbaum H, Kerber R, Kisslo J, Weyman AE, Nanda N, Popp RL, Sahn D, Schiller NB, Tajik AJ: Report of the American Society of Echocardiography Committee on Nomenclature and Standards: identification of myocardial wall segments. American Society of Echocardiography, Duke University Medical Center, 1982, 15 pp.

4. CLINICAL APPLICATIONS OF
2D TRANSESOPHAGEAL ECHOCARDIOGRAPHY

FROM DIAGNOSIS TO MONITORING

Echocardiography has been traditionally thought of in terms of diagnosis; the practical aspects of obtaining satisfactory images have precluded its use for continuous evaluation of cardiac function. Only with development of an esophageal transducer has interest developed in the use of echocardiography as a monitoring device. In this capacity, transesophageal echocardiography has found application in anesthetized patients, where it is used to monitor global left ventricular function and changes in regional function, which may be indicative of ischemia. For certain operative procedures, transesophageal echocardiography is useful for the detection and localization of intracardiac air, or for definition of intracardiac anatomy. Occasionally in critical care settings where surgical bandages or other impediments preclude the use of transthoracic transducers, the esophageal transducer may provide the means to accomplish cardiac imaging.

MONITORING FOR ISCHEMIA AND INFARCTION: AN
INTRODUCTION TO WALL MOTION ABNORMALITIES

In 1935, Tennant and Wiggers reported that ligation of a coronary artery produced an almost immediate failure of contraction in the ischemic area of the myocardium. In the open–chested animal, they observed that the heart muscle supplied by the ligated coronary artery first contracted poorly, then became immobile, and subsequently appeared to bulge during systole [1]. The occurrence of abnormal myocardial contraction was thus established as a sensitive marker of myocardial ischemia. Many investigators have since examined the relationship between myocardial perfusion and regional contraction [2–7]. In recent years, 2D echocardiography has provided a practical tool for the detection of ischemia and infarction both in research and clinical use. "Wall motion abnormality" is a nonspecific term applied to a segment or area of myocardium that is contracting or relaxing abnormally. Thus, wall motion abnormalities can occur in either systole or diastole, but systolic wall motion abnormalities have been more thoroughly investigated. The left ventricle is expected to thicken in systole, such that the ventricular cavity becomes smaller, and expels the stroke volume. With angiography, this motion is seen by opacification of the ventricular cavity so that endocardial motion is perceived, but not wall thickening. With echocardiography, both the endocardial and epicardial borders of the ventricular wall are seen so that both the endocardial motion and the wall thickening can be observed. Furthermore, by repositioning the ultrasound transducer, multiple cross-sectional views of the ventricle can be examined; whereas, with angiography, a profile view of the injected radiopaque dye is obtained in one or two views only, and more detailed examination requires several injections of dye and further x-ray exposure.

Several terms are in use to describe normal and abnormal wall motion: in describing 2D images, it is generally enough to describe wall motion as normal, hypokinetic, akinetic, or dyskinetic. Whereas hypokinesia and dyskinesia may be described as mild or severe, akinesia should not be similarly graded, since the term refers to the absence of movement. Notice that all these terms are generally referring to endocardial movement, and do not describe specifically systolic wall thickening, which is sometimes more difficult to appreciate from the image.

Terminology

Synergy describes a normally contracting ventricle.
Asynergy refers to abnormal contraction.
Asyneresis is a term also used to mean abnormal contraction.
Synchrony and *asynchrony* refer to the temporal sequence of con-

traction; when all parts of the myocardium contract at the same time, there is synchronous contraction. If some segments contract before others, there is asynchronous contraction.

Hypokinesia describes a weak contraction, not as vigorous as normally contracting myocardium.

Akinesia describes nonmoving myocardium; an area which fails to contract at all.

Dyskinesia refers to bulging of the myocardium during systole, such as occurs with a ventricular aneurysm.

Mechanism

The occurrence of wall motion abnormalities immediately following the onset of ischemia results from tissue hypoxia. Without oxygen, the production of ATP from ADP fails, the regulatory function of ATP is impaired, regional acidosis develops, and the net effect is an impairment of calcium delivery to the contractile elements. These pathophysiologic changes cause no histologic changes in the cell unless 5–20 min of ischemia elapse. As ischemia is prolonged, irreversible cellular changes occur, involving most cells of an ischemic area after 60 min. Thus, contraction abnormalities may be reversible, corresponding with reversible ischemia, or may be irreversible, characterizing an infarcted area of myocardium.

In animal studies, it has been demonstrated that complete coronary occlusion is followed within 10–15 s by hypokinesia of the affected myocardium. This progresses to akinesia and dyskinesia after 30–60 s [3–5]. Similar observations have recently been made in patients undergoing coronary occlusion during balloon angioplasty [8]. With controlled, graded coronary stenosis, this relationship of hypokinesia, akinesia, and dyskinesia persists; i.e., as a coronary artery is progressively occluded, the initial regional wall motion abnormality is hypokinesia, appearing with approximately 50% reduction in coronary flow. Dyskinesia appears with 90%–95% reductions in flow. The onset of regional wall motion abnormalities is very much dependent on heart rate, appearing much earlier in the presence of tachycardia, as would be expected. Abnormalities of contraction, therefore, appear when myocardial oxygen demand exceeds supply, and occur concomitantly with evidence of myocardial lactate production [9, 10]. Short coronary occlusions of 100 s are followed by functional recovery within 45 s [11]. In fact, regional contraction following such an occlusion may demonstrate a transient overshoot phenomenon in temporal relationship to the reactive hyperemia and catecholamine release. As the regional flow returns to preocclusion levels, the regional contraction pattern also returns to baseline. The occurrence of a regional wall motion abnormality, whether due to infarction or ischemia, also has some effect on the rest of the myocardium, which can add confusion to the picture. Experimental work has shown that with acute coronary occlusion there is depression of myocardial function beyond the infarct zone, the magnitude of which is inversely related to the distance from the infarct area [3, 12, 13]. This is seen almost immediately following coronary occlusion, and is persistent. Depressed function in areas beyond the infarct zone occurs in the absence of any ST-segment changes or alterations in local perfusion [13]. Other authors have described apparent hyperkinesia, or enhanced, compensatory function in nonischemic areas [12, 14]. This discrepancy in results probably occurred because of different experimental techniques and factors affecting contractility, e.g., preload, catecholamines, anesthesia. The effect of regional ischemia on nonischemic tissue is probably in part attributable to a "tethering" effect. The myocardial fibers are interwoven, such that noncontracting fibers would be expected to impair the contraction of adjacent normal fibers. It is consistent with this mechanism that areas remote from an infarct are less impaired than fibers immediately adjacent. Restoration of coronary perfusion and recovery of cellular function account for the reversibility of wall motion abnormalities seen experimentally and in human subjects.

Although the onset of a regional wall motion abnormality occurs almost simultaneously with ischemia, the restoration of normal wall motion may lag behind restoration of myocardial perfusion to a variable degree. It has been shown, for example, that a 5-min coronary occlusion results in wall motion abnormalities that persist for 3 h [15]; a 15-min occlusion results in contraction abnormalities lasting for more than 6 h. This persistence of impaired contractile function in the presence of restored perfusion characterizes the "stunned myocardium" and makes it very difficult to assess by echocardiography the extent of myocardial infarction following a coronary occlusion. This was demonstrated by Wyatt and Meerbaum in dogs [16] in which a 3-h coronary occlusion was followed by 45 h of reperfusion. The echocardiographic extent of regional wall motion abnormality was compared with the extent of infarction by nitroblue tetrazolium staining. A lack of correlation was seen during the reperfusion phase with myocardial edema, but the correlation improved as myocardial edema and hyperemia resolved. Patients undergoing coronary angioplasty for acute myocardial infarction and patients undergoing cardiac surgery may exhibit reperfusion wall motion abnormalities. Estimates of viable and nonviable tissue made on the basis of echocardiographic images cannot be reliable in such patients [17]. The observed dysfunction is real, however, and may be helpful in guiding therapy to optimize cardiac performance and sustain the circulation.

Depression of myocardial function following infarction is due, therefore, to more than isolated regional dysfunction in the infarct zone alone. It is easy to see why 2D echocardiography would tend to overestimate the size of an infarct. Experimentally, wall thickening has been shown to delineate the extent of an infarct more precisely than endocardial motion [13, 18, 19]. Lieberman and coworkers [18] also noted that an infarct involving less than 20% of the wall thickness exhibited reduced wall thickening, whereas more than 20% involvement caused wall thinning. There was, however, no significant augmentation in the severity of systolic thinning as the extent of transmural infarction increased from 21% to 100%. Generally speaking, the extent of severe wall motion abnormality serves to mark the extent of an infarction, with noninfarcted adjacent zones exhibiting milder hypokinesia only.

Echocardiographic localization of myocardial infarction

Generally, the anterior wall of the left ventricle and 75% of the interventricular septum are supplied by the left anterior descending coronary artery (LAD), the lateral wall by the circumflex coronary or branches of the LAD, and the posterior wall by the right coronary artery. The occurrence and location of regional wall motion abnormalities with myocardial infarction were examined by Heger and coworkers, who found segmental wall motion abnormalities in all of 37 patients with documented myocardial infarction. They described the location of the wall motion abnormalities in relation to the ECG changes [20]. The left ventricle was divided into nine segments including four at the midpapillary muscle level (figure 4-1). Of the 37 patients, 29 had more than one segment exhibiting a wall motion abnormality. The most frequently involved segments were those seen in the midpapillary muscle short-axis view (nos. 5–8) and the apex (no. 9). All of 14 patients with anterior infarction by ECG had anterior wall asynergy by 2D echocardiography; 19 of the 20 patients with inferior infarction by ECG had posterior wall asynergy. Septal asynergy occurs frequently in association with anterior wall infarction because the left anterior descending coronary artery generally supplies

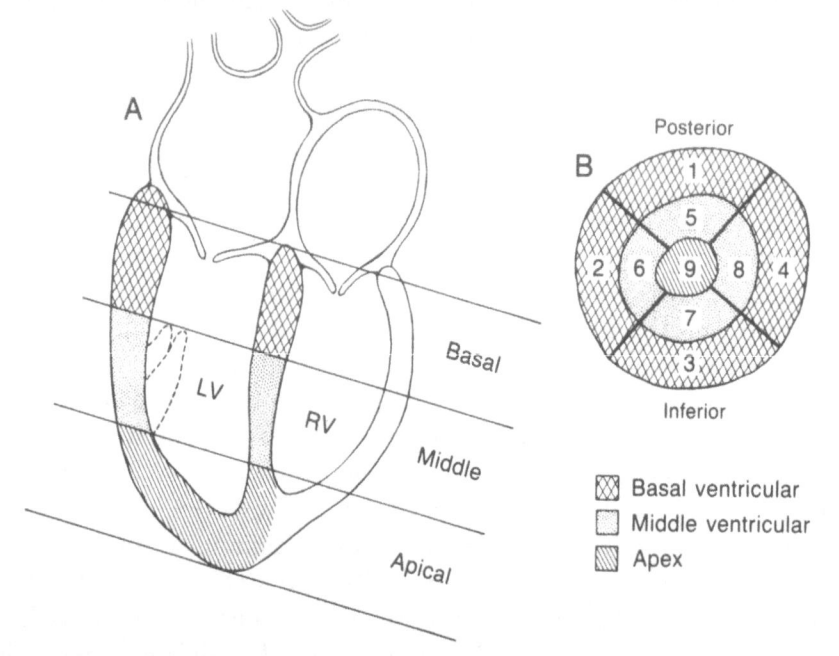

Figure 4-1. Segmental division of left ventricular wall: (A) long-axis view and (B) as seen from the apex.

both regions. Septal asynergy has been used as a marker of stenosis in this coronary artery [21]. Echocardiographic studies of patients with coronary artery disease confirm a high incidence of wall motion abnormalities [21, 22]. Corya and coworkers found abnormal wall motion in 89% of patients with Q-wave evidence of infarction by ECG; 61% of patients with coronary artery disease but no evidence of infarction by ECG also had abnormal regional wall motion [21].

Relative sensitivity of regional wall motion and electrocardiography for the detection of ischemia

The surface ECG shows ST-segment elevation at about 30–60 s following coronary occlusion. Therefore, provided an appropriate lead is monitored, it should be possible to identify myocardial infarction almost as quickly by ECG as by 2D echocardiography. Of more interest, however, is the occurrence of ischemia without infarction, which is likely to occur much more frequently in clinical practice. In the experimental animal, hypokinesia affecting an ischemic area occurs routinely before ECG changes appear, if they appear at all [10]. Waters and coworkers found that hypokinesia appeared first at approximately 50% reduction in coronary flow, and ECG changes developed at approximately 75% reduction in flow [10]. Similar results have been reported elsewhere [23, 24]. Comparison of contractile function and ECG changes in the epicardium and endocardium further reveal that contraction abnormalities appear first in the subendocardium and, again, these precede ST changes from endocardial leads, which themselves appear long before surface lead ECG changes. It is not surprising that ischemia should manifest itself initially in the subendocardium, which is known to be at greatest risk with coronary stenosis. Smith and coworkers [25] compared surface electrocardiography and 2D echocardiography for detection of ischemia in 50 anesthetized patients with known coronary artery disease. Of the fifty patients, 24 developed new segmental wall motion abnormalities intraoperatively, but only six developed ST-segment changes. ST-segment changes were always accompanied by wall motion abnormalities that developed before or simultaneously with ST-segment changes. Of the three patients who developed perioperative myocardial infarctions, only one had intraoperative ST-segment changes, whereas all had persistent new wall motion abnormalities. This clinical study corroborates the animal studies indicating that the sensitivity and specificity of regional wall motion abnormalities for the detection of ischemia are clearly superior to the electrocardiogram. It would appear that transesophageal 2D echocardiography could find widespread application for the monitoring of patients at risk for ischemia.

Intraoperative detection of regional wall motion abnormalities

Clinical, qualitative, real-time examination of 2D images for segmental wall motion abnormalities requires that one develop the habit of examining each segment in turn for wall thickening and inward motion during systole (figure 4–2). The midpapillary short-axis view, which includes segments of myocardium representing all three coronary arteries, is the best single view to monitor. If the patient's coronary anatomy is known from angiography, however, those myocardial segments known to be at risk for ischemia can be selected. The appearance of significant wall motion abnormalities is usually obvious, but subtle changes may be difficult to pinpoint unless images can be compared over time. Some echocardiographs allow up to four images to be recalled to the video screen for this purpose. Anesthesiologists unfamiliar with 2D echocardiography may question their ability to recognize wall motion abnormalities on the video

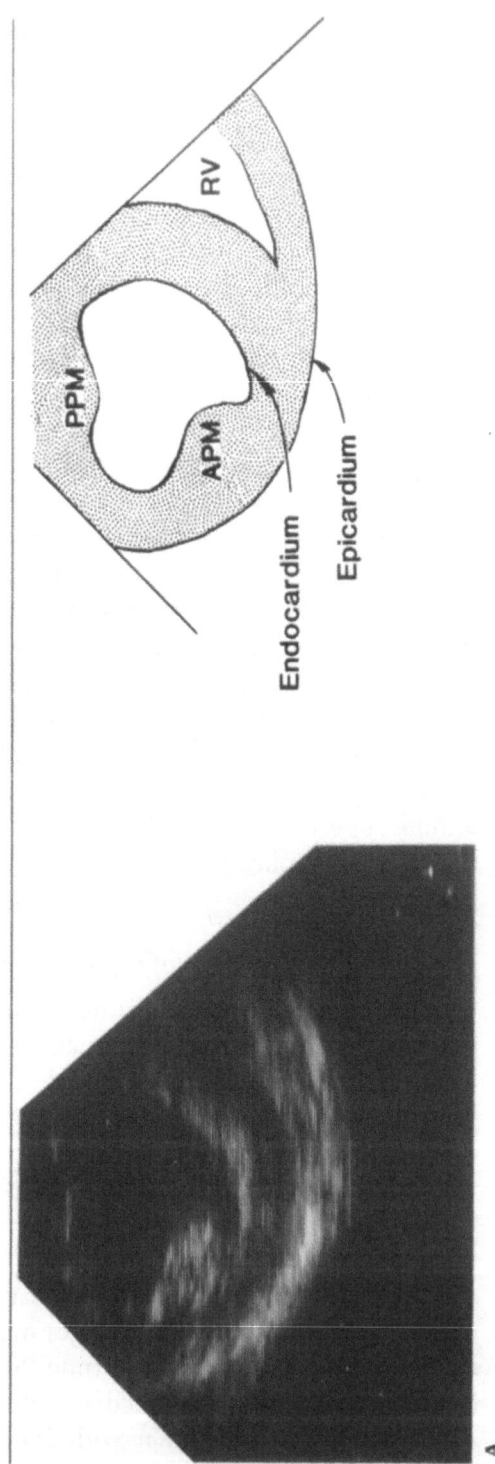

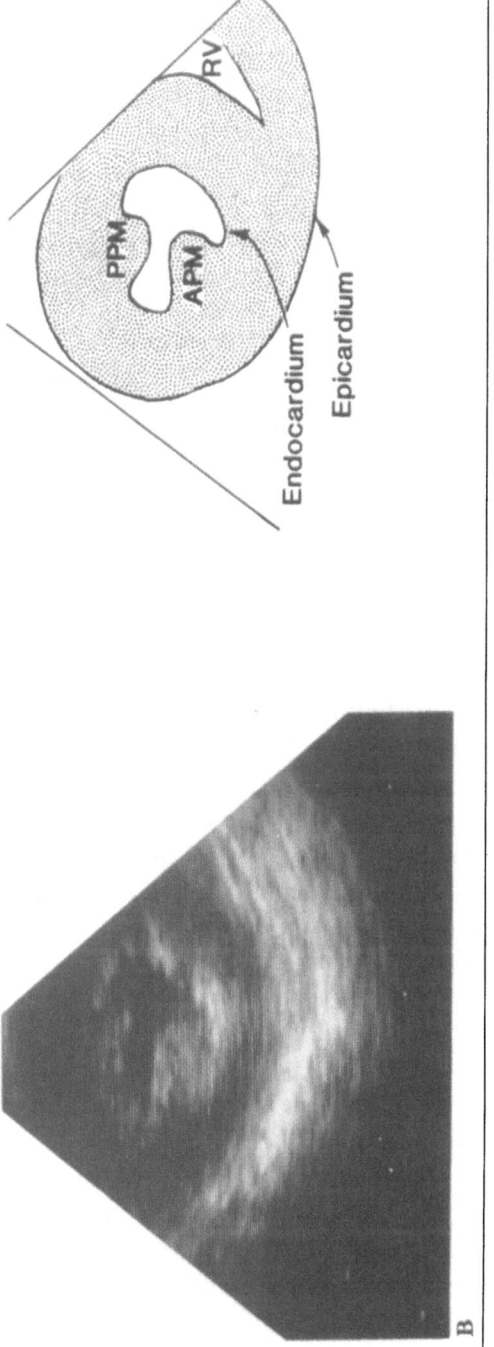

Figure 4–2. Short-axis view at papillary muscle levels, left ventricle: (A) diastole and (B) systole. RV = right ventricle, PPM = posterior papillary muscle, and APM = anterior papillary muscle.

image, but the authors have found this skill is easily learned [26]. We took a group of 53 clinicians, including anesthesiologists, nurse anesthetists, and anesthesia residents, and gave them 20 min of instruction about transesophageal echocardiography and the recognition of regional wall motion abnormalities. With this background, they were then asked to grade regional wall motion for 12 videotape recordings, and their scores were compared with those of four trained observers. The 53 clinicians correctly identified 95% of the regional wall motion abnormalities. They correctly assessed 62% of the normally contracting regions, with the incorrect responses (38%) being most frequently hypokinesia (32%), the mildest grade of abnormality.

Regional wall motion abnormalities and open-heart surgery

Echocardiographic studies of patients undergoing open-heart surgery, intraoperatively and postoperatively, have indicated that some wall motion abnormalities may not necessarily indicate ischemia or infarction. Septal wall motion abnormalities following aortic and mitral valve replacements have been reported by several investigators [27, 28]. There is no clear explanation for this; the aortic and mitral valves are anchored onto tissue immediately adjacent to the septum, however, and a tethering effect may contribute to this observed hypokinesia or dyskinesia. Vignola and coworkers [29] studied septal motion prospectively in 45 patients before and after cardiac surgery, finding septal wall motion abnormalities in 31 of the 40 patients who required cardiopulmonary bypass, and in none of the five patients not requiring cardiopulmonary bypass. It was noted that, of the 40 patients undergoing cardiopulmonary bypass, potassium cardioplegia was used in 18 of 31 patients developing septal wall motion abnormalities and in one of nine patients having normal septal motion. Righetti and coworkers [30] followed 40 patients postoperatively after coronary artery bypass grafting and found abnormal septal motion present prior to hospital discharge. Using a different system of image analysis, Force and coworkers [31] found no septal motion abnormalities in 15 patients undergoing coronary artery bypass surgery. Some of these conflicting results undoubtedly occur because of different techniques, images, and methods of analysis. In particular, analysis of endocardial motion can be confounded by movement of the heart as a whole within the chest, and by pericardiotomy (see chapter 5). The use of systolic wall thickening for analysis should help to overcome these difficulties.

Guiding therapy by regional wall motion

Clinically, patients with diffuse coronary artery disease have several areas of potentially compromised perfusion that can be altered by drug therapy, and these areas may be at risk from the effects of tachycardia or coronary spasm. Several investigators have compared the effects of drugs on ischemic and nonischemic myocardium by echocardiography [14, 32]. Nitroglycerin and propranolol improve regional function during acute coronary occlusion; isoproterenol may cause an initial improvement followed by later impairment of function. Thus, efficacy of treatment can be instantaneously assessed in clinical management. Drug interventions have been used in conjunction with echocardiography to identify areas of reversible ischemia that may benefit from coronary bypass grafting. Approximately 60% of patients with coronary artery disease exhibit regional wall motion abnormalities at rest [21, 22], a proportion of which can be improved by nitroglycerin and represent areas of chronic ischemia in viable myocardium. Likewise, regional wall motion abnormalities can be uncovered by exercise, or by raising the heart rate with pacing, forming the basis for "stress echocardiography" in the diagnosis of coronary artery disease.

Intraoperative monitoring of global left ventricular function

Using the same papillary muscle level short-axis view that is monitored for regional wall motion abnormalities, the 2D image provides information about the size of the left ventricle and its contractility. 2D images have been used, therefore, to measure preload, afterload, and various derived parameters describing contractility in a quantitative fashion (see chapter 5). Computer software designed to allow these calculations to be made in a timely fashion is gradually becoming available to the clinician. Qualitative assessment is generally used in the operating room and is prone to the inaccuracies of any subjective evaluation. Nevertheless, with a little experience, the practicing anesthesiologist can find the 2D images very helpful in assessing cardiac function. It is predictable that, with provision of on-line quantitative information from transesophageal 2D echocardiography (TEE), the indication for a pulmonary artery catheter may be obviated in most patients presently requiring them for intraoperative management.

Preload

Left ventricular preload or the volume of blood in the left ventricle at end-diastole is presently assessed at best by measurement of the mean left atrial pressure (LAP) or pulmonary capillary wedge pressure (PCWP). Clinically the assessment of preload is made difficult when the pressure–volume relationship is altered by the stiffness of the left ventricle, or its compliance. Since diseased ventricles often have poor compliance, it is in exactly the patients most in need of careful hemo-dynamic management that the assessment of preload by pressure measurement is most inaccurate. With 2D-TEE we now have the opportunity to measure preload more directly. Although end-diastolic volume can be calculated from multiple views, a single short-axis end-diastolic area (EDA) serves very well, and is normally 6–14 cm^2 at the midpapillary muscle level. Haendchen (see Ch. 5) found the mean EDA in 14 normal subjects to be 11.7 cm^2 at midpapillary muscle level, varying from 16.3 cm^2 at the mitral valve level to 9.8 cm^2 at a low left ventricle level. The normal variation in EDA at different cross-sectional levels in the same subject emphasizes the need to use the same level for serial monitoring of preload. Dubroff and coworkers [33] studied EDA with a sterile, on-the-heart 2D echo transducer in patients undergoing cardiac surgery, noting that correction of aortic regurgitation was accompanied by an immediate decrease in EDA, and found that this was not observed with valve replacement for mitral disease or aortic stenosis. Roizen and coworkers [34] studied 24 patients undergoing aortic occlusion for reconstructive vascular surgery and noted significant increases in EDA with aortic occlusion, often in the absence of corre-sponding increases in PCWP.

Afterload/wall stress

Afterload on the left ventricle has always represented a difficult quantity to measure clinically, since it must be inferred from the systolic blood pressure. Afterload is really of consequence because it relates to the stress imposed on the left ventricular wall and hence to the myocardial oxygen consumption. An on-line index of wall stress would therefore provide the clinician with moment-to-moment infor-mation about the myocardial oxygen consumption of his patient. At the same time, the presence or absence of regional wall motion abnor-malities indicates the adequacy or inadequacy of the myocardial oxygen supply. Wall stress is calculated by the formula:

$$\text{wall stress} = \frac{\text{pressure} \times \text{radius}}{\text{wall thickness}}$$

2D-TEE images with the addition of a ventricular pressure measurement can provide the means to calculate wall stress. For peak stress, it has been shown that cuff systolic blood pressure is very adequate [35], provided that there is no aortic valvular disease. Roizen and coworkers [34] found that, with supraceliac occlusion of the aorta, mean systemic arterial pressure increased 54%, and was accompanied by an increase in end-systolic area of 69%. Occlusion of the aorta more distally was accompanied by only minor increases in mean arterial pressure and end-systolic area. Wall stress was not calculated, but it is clear that a marked increase occurred with supraceliac aortic occlusion. The consequence of substantial increases in myocardial oxygen consumption is reflected by the occurrence of ischemia in 92% of patients undergoing supraceliac aortic occlusion in this study.

EVALUATION OF CARDIAC ANATOMY

The visualization of cardiac structures with 2D-TEE offers some specific advantages in patients undergoing intracardiac surgery. The mitral, tricuspid, and aortic valves are well seen with TEE, the posteriorly situated mitral valve being better seen by TEE than by transthoracic echocardiography (figure 4-3). In addition to the valve leaflets, the chordae tendineae and papillary muscles can be identified quite easily, in both short- and long-axis views. Prosthetic valves can also be evaluated intraoperatively for mobility. The use of contrast further extends the use of 2D-TEE. Indocyanine green dye, saline, or 5% dextrose injected rapidly can all serve as contrast material, even when injected through a peripheral vein. The contrast effect is generated by microbubbles in the injectate, and thus substances with a relatively high surface tension such as indocyanine green dye hold bubbles better and make better contrast agents.

Intraoperatively, contrast can often be injected directly into the right atrium or ventricle via a central venous pressure line, or an indwelling pulmonary artery catheter port. In this way, the presence of right-to-left shunts can be identified by the appearance of contrast in the left atrium and ventricle, and the competence of the tricuspid valve can be assessed by looking for appearance of contrast in the right atrium following a right ventricular injection. Although less obvious, echocardiographers have noted a "negative contrast" effect

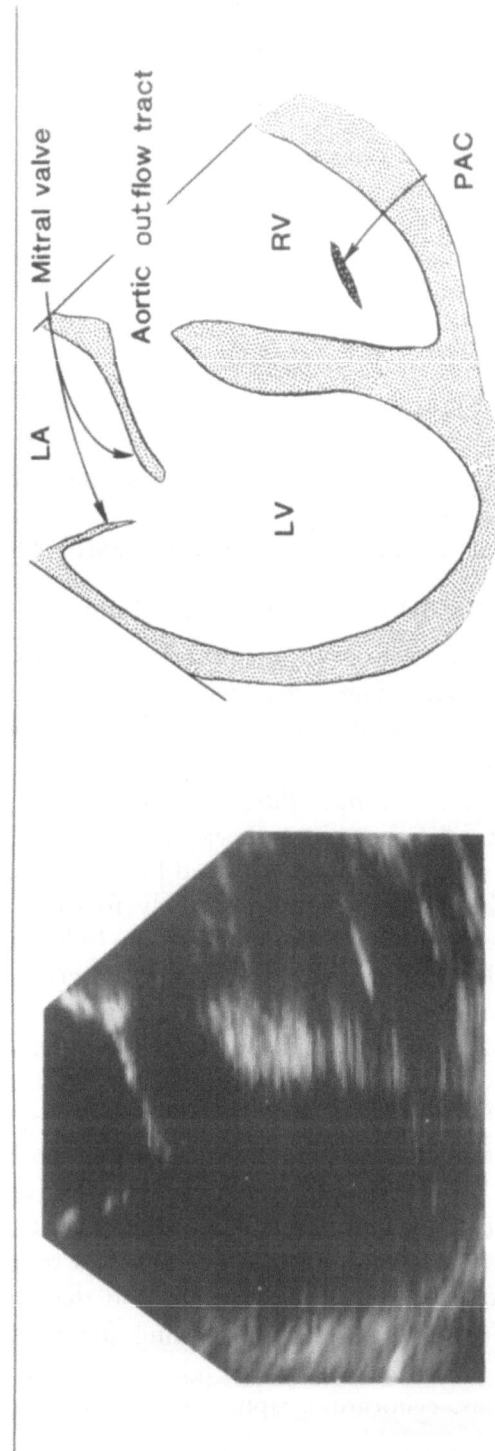

Figure 4-3. Normal mitral valve; long-axis view: LV = left ventricle, LA = left atrium, RV = right ventricle, and PAC = pulmonary artery catheter (echo artifact seen in right ventricle).

helpful for the identification of left-to-right shunts, using a right-sided injection [36]. In the presence of significant left-to-right shunt at the atrial level, for example, opacification of the right atrium by a contrast injection may be incomplete because of shunted blood entering the right atrium from the left atrium through an atrial septal defect. An echo-free defect then appears in the contrast-filled right atrium and is termed a negative contrast effect. Other maneuvers can be used to demonstrate left-to-right shunting, or at least the presence of a communication between the right and left sides; in the anesthetized patient, the delivery of a prolonged inspiration during mechanical ventilation, followed by abrupt release of intrathoracic pressure, causes a transient gradient of pressure from the right to the left atrium as the right atrium fills with blood and the left atrium remains relatively empty. Contrast injected into the right atrium during the one or two cardiac cycles following the prolonged inspiration may then cross an atrial septal defect that normally shunts only left-to-right. The successful delivery of contrast into the left heart has also been reported with injection of contrast through the distal port of a wedged pulmonary artery catheter. Passage of microbubbles through the pulmonary circulation has been well documented; with administration of a pulmonary vasodilator bubbles up to 130 microns in diameter can pass [37]. However, left-sided contrast injections are more reliably achieved by direct injection into the cardiac apex, or into an indwelling left atrial catheter. Eguaras and coworkers [38] employed contrast (5% dextrose) for evaluation of mitral and aortic regurgitation intraoperatively, using a sterile on-the-heart transducer. Contrast was injected into the left ventricle for mitral regurgitation and into the ascending aorta for aortic regurgitation. The degree of regurgitation estimated by echocardiography correlated very well with preoperative cineangiographic estimates. Thus, contrast echocardiography provides additional information about directional blood flow within the heart which complements the structural information provided by 2D images. With increasing efforts to repair rather than replace valves, the need for intraoperative evaluation has markedly increased. Another technological development for the identification of blood flow and velocity has now become available in conjunction with 2D echocardiography: Doppler echocardiography uses the principle of frequency shifts to characterize blood flow. Thus, pulses of ultrasound can be directed from the transducer into a "sample volume" of blood identified on the 2D image. The direction and velocity of blood flow in this or other sample volumes can be characterized (see chapter 6). Doppler information can be presented as aural signals, and also graphically as a time-interval histogram in conjunction with an M-mode echocardiogram. More recently, Doppler information is being presented in a color-coded form combined with 2D echocardiograms, providing instantaneous visualization of intracardiac blood flow on the 2D image. This color-flow mapping technology, with an esophageal transducer, should provide for the first time a convenient, noninvasive, real-time method of assessing cardiac integrity intraoperatively. The potential application in patients with congenital heart disease is enormous. However, the size of the transesophageal probe will have to be reduced for most pediatric patients.

DETECTION OF INTRACARDIAC AIR

Intracardiac air is easily seen with echocardiography, and this characteristic has prompted the use of transesophageal echocardiography for the detection of air during neurosurgical procedures in the sitting position and in cardiac surgery. Unfortunately air cannot be easily quantified by echocardiography and most investigators have attempted to grade the appearance of air in a semi-quantitative way. Microbubbles are identified as small, oblong, highly mobile, echodense particles appearing on the 2D video frame; the amount of air has been graded from 0 to 3, where 0 = no particles, 1 = fewer than 5/frame, 2 = 10–25/frame, and 3 = too numerous to count [39, 40].

Cucchiara and coworkers [41] studied the use of TEE to detect and localize air embolism, comparing it with the use of precordial Doppler in neurosurgical patients. In 15 patients, three emboli were detected by Doppler. All were visualized with TEE by the appearance of air in the right atrium. An additional two questionable air emboli by Doppler were unequivocally demonstrated by TEE. In one patient, air was seen to enter the left atrium, presumably via a patent foramen ovale. No neurologic sequelae developed postoperatively. In neurosurgical patients, 2D-TEE promises to be at least as sensitive as precordial Doppler, and additionally can localize the air to the right or left side of the heart.

In open-heart surgery, elimination of air from the left side of the heart is always a concern. Rodrigas and coworkers [39] recorded 2D images in 79 patients before and after cardiopulmonary bypass, using a hand-held sterile transducer applied directly on the heart. Microbubbles were detected in 49% of patients after bypass, and judged moderate or severe in 25%. Bubbles were detected more commonly in patients undergoing valve replacements or atrial septal defect repairs in whom the left side of the heart was open to air. Evidence of air persisted for as long as 60 min after cardiopulmonary bypass. Neurologic or psychologic testing was not performed in these patients; however, no patient developed a clinically apparent neurologic injury. These observations were corroborated more recently by Topol and coworkers [40], who recorded 2D images of the heart in 82 patients undergoing cardiac surgery, using 2D-TEE. Microbubbles were detected in 41% of patients after cardiopulmonary bypass (figure 4-4). Again, intracardiac procedures were associated with significantly more appearances of microbubbles (74%) than with extracardiac procedures, such as coronary artery bypass grafting (12%). No patient developed a focal neurologic deficit and serial neurologic examinations did not indicate any association between severity of microbubbles and neurologic outcome. However, detailed prospective neuropsychiatric testing was not done in this study. Neurologic injury can be quite subtle following open-heart surgery [42, 43]. Since 2D echocardiography detects very small bubbles 2–100 μ in diameter that may be cleared from the circulation without impairing tissue perfusion, it is quite conceivable that the echocardiographic appearance of air should not be associated with gross neurologic deficit. However, more detailed prospective studies of neuropsychiatric function may be necessary to define the significance of intracardiac air during surgery. Topol and coworkers [40] noted that attempts to evacuate air manually from the left ventricle were never completely successful, but some improvement could be demonstrated echocardiographically by a reduction in the amount of microbubble echoes.

Clearly the ability to quantify air by 2D echocardiography would have major clinical significance. Likewise the ability to localize air to a right- or left-sided cardiac chamber carries additional importance. Several authors have noted that the incidence of probe-patent foramen ovale is 20%–35% in the adult population and, with elevation of the right atrial pressure relative to the left atrial pressure, the potential for paradoxical air embolism exists.

Atrial septal defects

Atrial septal defects are identified on the 2D image by the appearance of a defect in the echo-dense line representing the interatrial septum. Artifactual defects are sometimes created by echo "dropout," which tends to occur with a structure lying parallel to the ultrasound beam. For this reason, transthoracic images are often plagued by echo dropout in the atrial septum, giving rise to a high incidence of false-positive readings for this lesion [44]. By the transesophageal route, however, the atrial septum lies in a plane more perpendicular to the ultrasound beam, and can be fully visualized by slight adjustments in transducer position within the esophagus. Hanrath and coworkers [45] compared the value of 2D-TEE and conventional transthoracic echocardiography for the identification of secundum atrial septal defects in 20 patients. Of these patients, 19 had satisfactory images by 2D-TEE and the atrial defect was reliably identified; 18 patients had satisfactory images using a transthoracic approach, but in only ten could the defect be identified. Quantitative assessment of the size of the defect correlated very well with direct measurement at the time of surgery. In addition, contrast studies (10 ml agitated saline injected via a peripheral vein) were performed to assess interatrial shunt. Contrast (microbubbles) was detected in the left atrium in 100% patients by TEE, and in 78% of the same patients imaged transthoracically. A negative contrast effect in the right atrium was noted in 37% patients by TEE and 11% with transthoracic images. In an additional 30 patients with no atrial septal defect, TEE images specifically excluded this lesion. Similar findings were reported by Reifart and coworkers [46], who found that 2D-TEE had a sensitivity of 95% and a specificity of 100% for the detection of atrial septal defects in 20 patients. By comparison, transthoracic 2D echocardiography had a sensitivity of 61% and a specificity of 88% (figure 4-5).

Left atrial disorders

Miscellaneous reports have appeared in the literature concerning the imaging of left atrial pathology. Since the left atrium lies posteriorly, it is the cardiac chamber least well visualized from the chest wall. Hence it is not surprising that the transesophageal approach offers better imaging. Two published reports concern the definition of left atrial myxomas by 2D-TEE [47, 48]. Thier and coworkers [48] found that transesophageal imaging allowed definition of cysts within the myxoma that could not be seen transthoracically. The same group has reported two patients in whom 2D-TEE allowed the definitive diagnosis of cor triatriatum to be made [49]. In this rare condition, a fenestrated membranous structure divides the left atrium and obstructs pulmonary venous drainage into the left ventricle, functionally mimicking mitral stenosis. The high-resolution images obtained with TEE permit definition of such structures.

Mitral valve disease

The mitral valve can generally be fairly well seen from the chest wall. However, TEE may offer some advantage. Schlüter and coworkers [50] found that TEE correctly diagnosed rupture of the chordae tendineae of the mitral leaflets in ten patients (figure 4-6). Transthoracic M-mode echocardiography diagnosed only three and 2D seven. In addition, a distinctive coiled echo structure was apparent in the left atrium during systole by TEE; the investigators suggested that this represented the free chorda tendinea recoiling into the left atrium. The resolution of transthoracic images has presumably been inadequate to define this delicate structure. The same group of investigators has examined the sensitivity and specificity of transesophageal pulsed Doppler echocardiography in the detection of mitral regurgitation [51]. They examined six patients with competent mitral valves and 12 with angiographically proven mild-to-moderate mitral regurgitation. The normal patients were found to have competent valves by both techniques. With valvular incompetence, mitral regurgitation was detected in 100% of patients with transesophageal Doppler but in only 58% of patients studied with transthoracic Doppler. The investigators attributed this advantage of the transesophageal approach to four factors: (a) the absence of anatomic obstacles between the transducer and the heart, (b) nearly parallel alignment of the ultrasound beam with the direction of blood flow, (c) the use of high pulse repetition frequencies, and (d) detection of localized regurgitant jets by left atrial scanning (see chapter 6). With mitral stenosis, the valve leaflets characteristically appear thickened and immobile. The left atrium is typically enlarged and the left ventricle relatively small (figure 4-7).

Aortic disease

Immediately adjacent to the esophagus lies the aorta. In situations where angiography is difficult to accomplish and/or transthoracic imaging is not possible, 2D-TEE may be helpful. Borner and colleagues have reported a patient with type-III aortic dissection that could not be identified with transthoracic imaging but only with TEE [52].

As cardiologists become more familiar with the idea of transesophageal imaging, it is likely to find routine application in patients who cannot be imaged transthoracically, as it has in some centers in Europe.

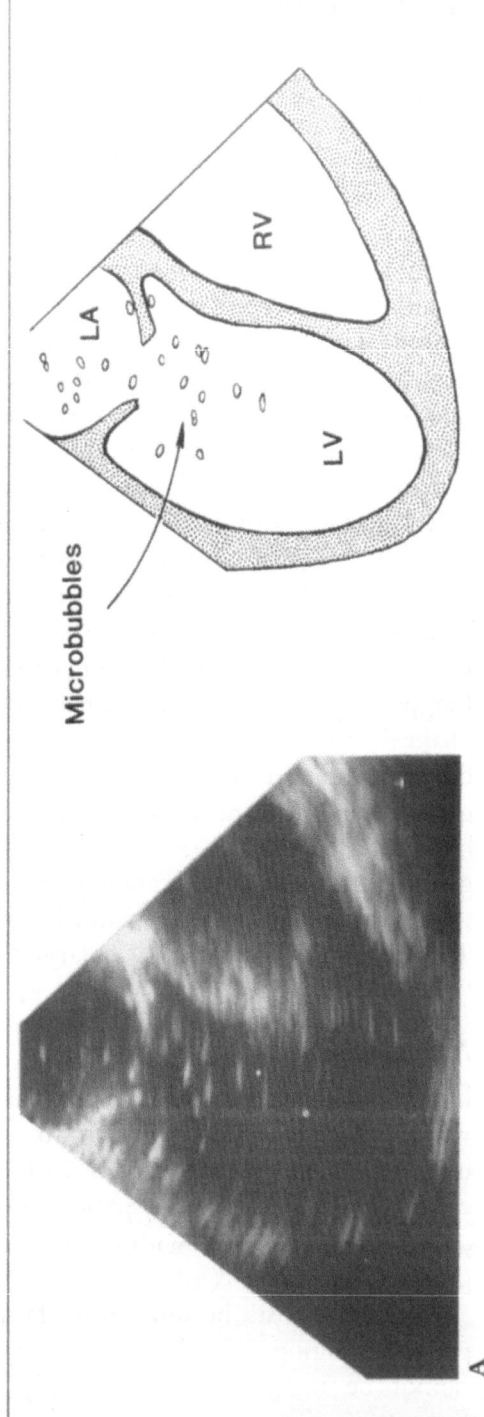

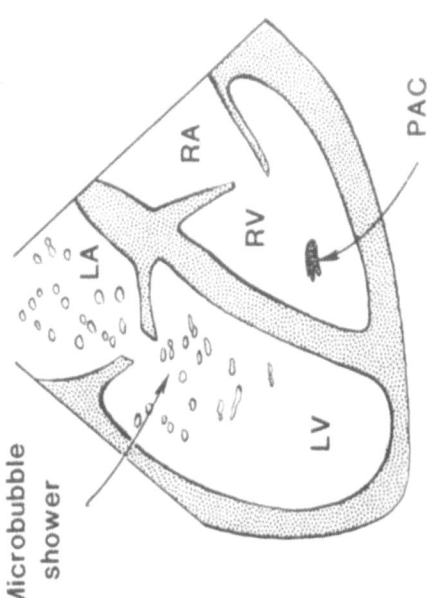

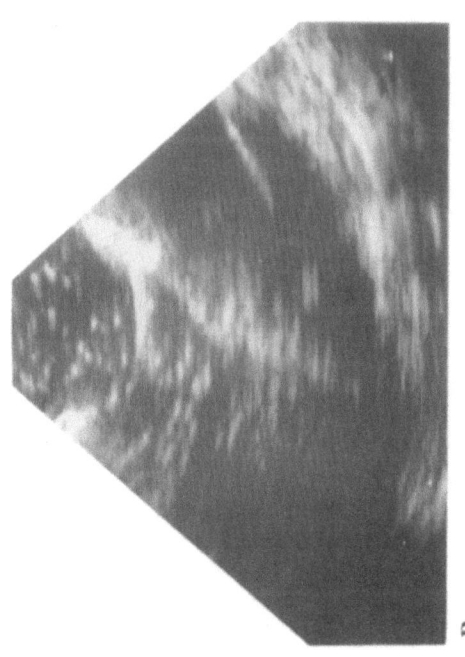

Figure 4-4. Intracardiac air microbubbles seen in the left atrium and left ventricle following aortic valve replacement: (A) grade 2, (10–25 particles/frame), and (B) grade 3 (too numerous to count).

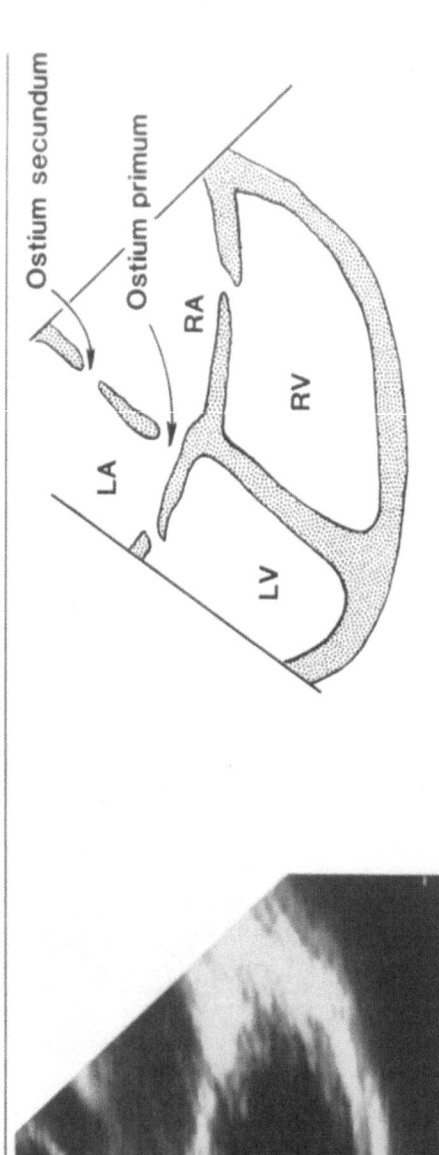

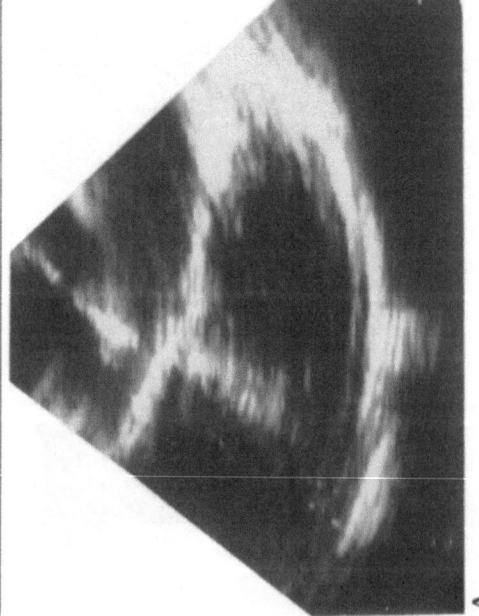

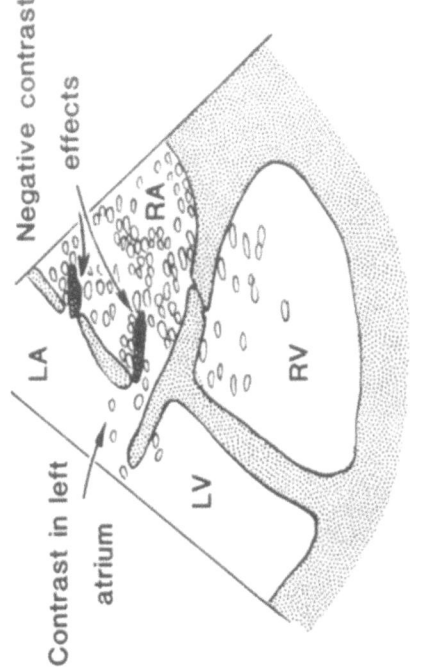

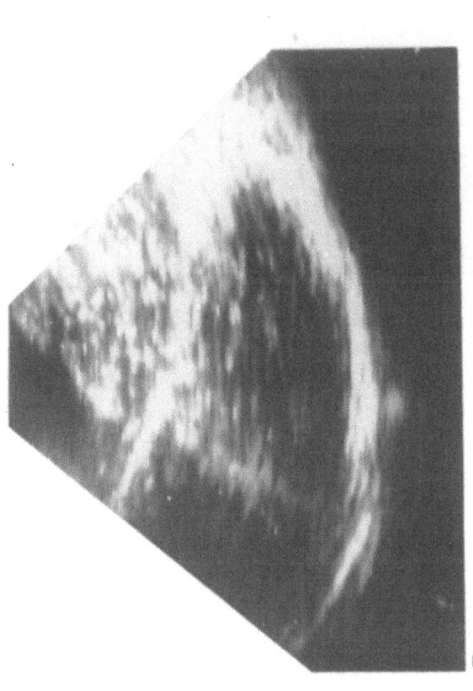

Figure 4-5. Atrial septal defects: (A) This patient had both ostium primum and ostium secundum defects, with a cleft mitral valve. (B) Contrast opacifies the right atrium with some crossing into the left atrium and left ventricle. Jets of blood from the left atrium create negative contrast effects in the right atrium. There is evidence of bidirectional shunting, therefore, in this patient.

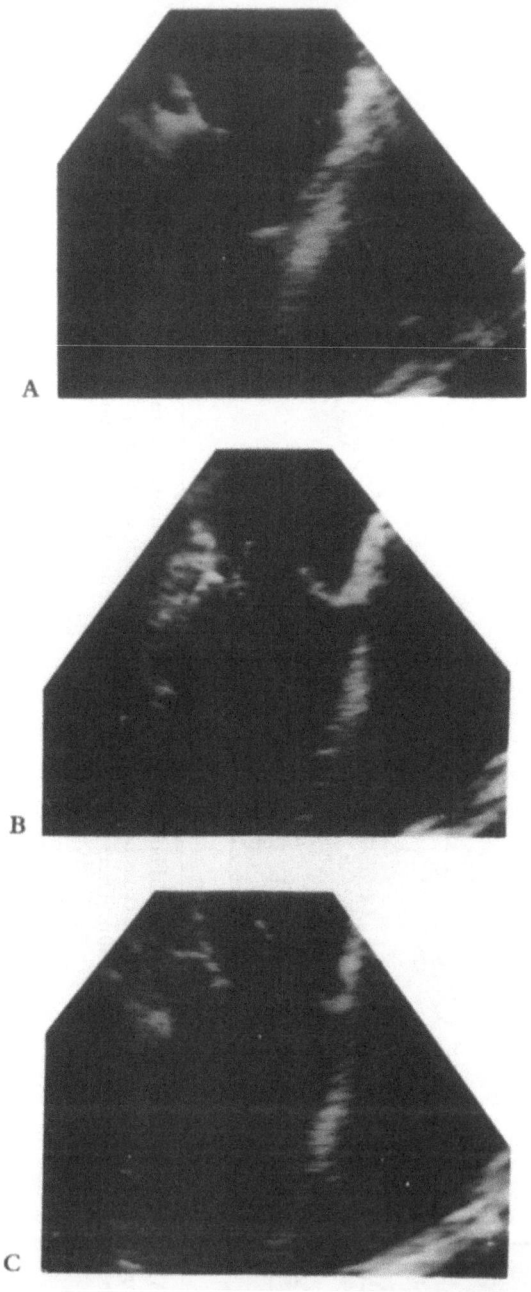

Figure 4-6. Flail anterior mitral leaflet due to a ruptured chorda tendinae: (A) diastole, (B) systole (coiled chorda), and (C) systole.

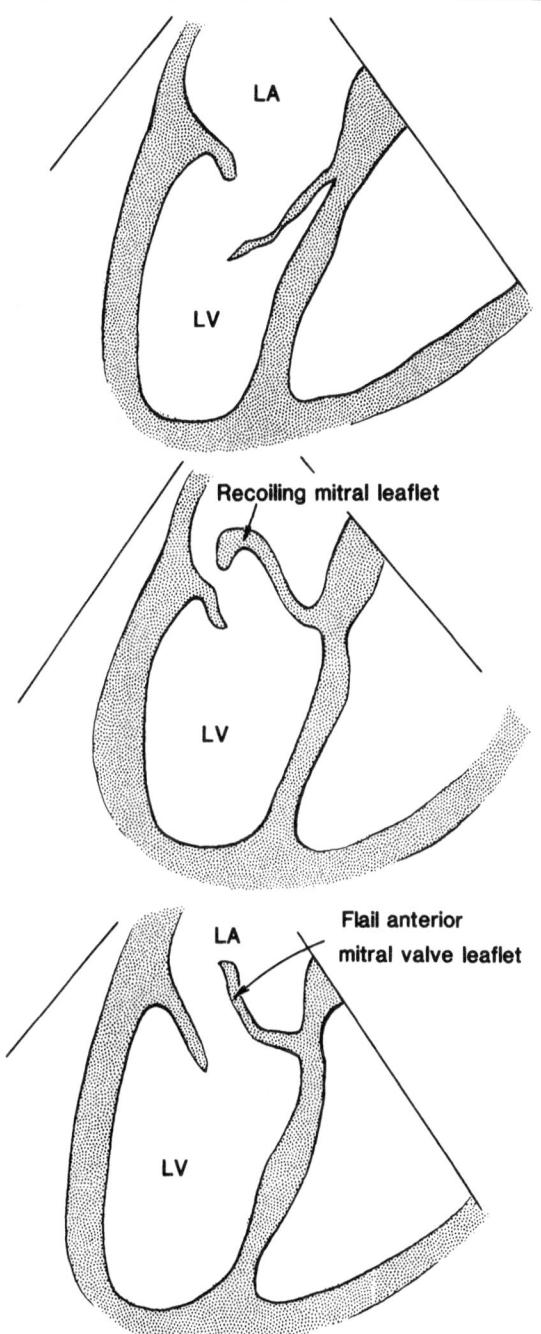

Recoiling mitral leaflet

Flail anterior
mitral valve leaflet

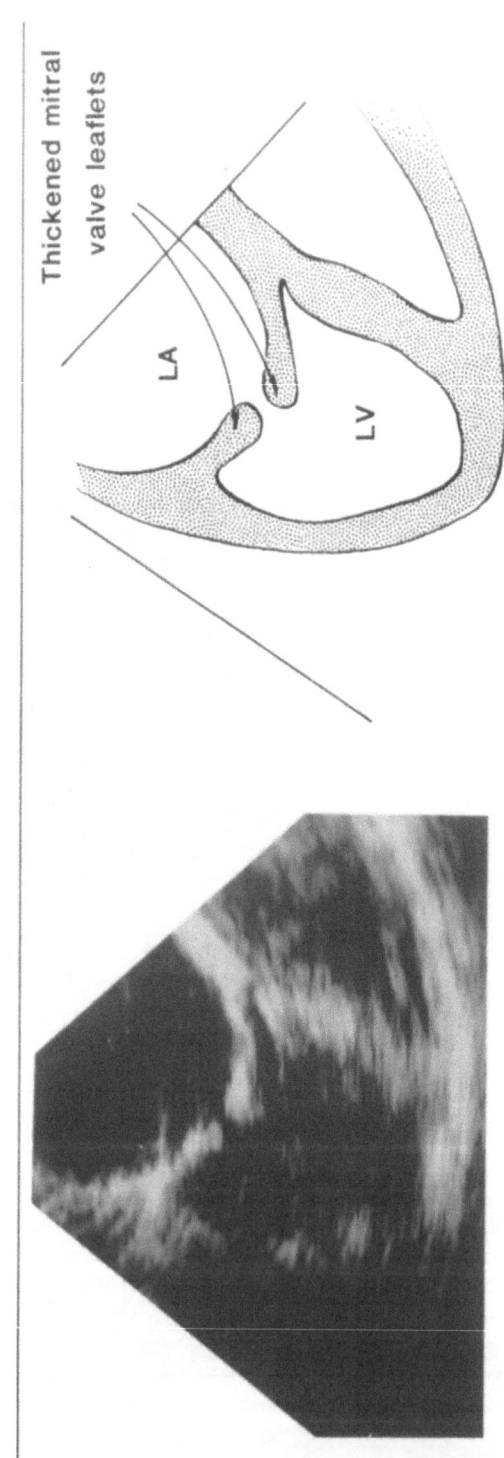

Figure 4-7. Mitral stenosis.

REFERENCES

1. Tennant R, Wiggers CJ: The effect of coronary occlusion on myocardial contraction. Am J Physiol 112:351–361, 1935.
2. Ross J, Franklin D: Analysis of regional myocardial function, dimensions, and wall thickness in the characterization of myocardial ischemia and infarction. Circulation [Suppl 1] 53:1-88-I-92, 1976.
3. Kerber RE, Marcus ML, Ehrhardt J, Wilson R, Abboud FM: Correlation between echocardiographically demonstrated segmental dyskinesis and regional myocardial perfusion. Circulation 52:1097–1104, 1975.
4. Battler A, Froelicher VF, Gallagher KP, Kemper WS, Ross J: Dissociation between regional myocardial dysfunction and ECG changes during ischemia in the conscious dog. Circulation 62:735–744, 1980.
5. Smith HJ, Kent KM, Epstein SE: Relationship between regional contractile function and S-T segment elevation after experimental coronary artery occlusion in the dog. Cardiovasc Res 12:444–448, 1978.
6. Vatner SF: Correlation between acute reductions in myocardial blood flow and function in conscious dogs. Circ Res 47:201–207, 1980.
7. Wyatt HL, Forrester JS, Tyberg JV, Goldner SE, Logan SE, Parmley WW, Swan HJC: Effect of graded reductions in regional coronary perfusion on regional and total cardiac function. Am J Cardiol 36:185–192, 1975.
8. Alam M, Khaja F, Brymer J, Marzelli M, Goldstein S: Echocardiographic evaluation of left ventricular function during coronary artery angioplasty. Am J Cardiol 57:20–25, 1986.
9. Massie BM, Botvinick EH, Brundage BH, Greenberg B, Shames D, Gelberg H: Relationship of regional myocardial perfusion to segmental wall motion: a physiological basis for understanding the presence of reversibility of asynergy. Circulation 58:1154–1163, 1978.
10. Waters DD, Da Luz P, Wyatt HL, Swan HJC, Forrester JS: Early changes in regional and global left ventricular function induced by graded reductions in regional coronary perfusion. Am J Cardiol 39:537–543, 1977.
11. Pagani M, Vatner SF, Baig H, Braunwald E: Initial myocardial adjustments to brief periods of ischemia and reperfusion in the conscious dog. Circ Res 43:83–92, 1978.
12. Wyatt HL, Forrester JS, Da Luz PL, Diamond GA, Chagrasulis R, Swan HJC: Functional abnormalities in nonoccluded regions of myocardium after experimental coronary occlusion. Am J Cardiol 37:366–372, 1976.
13. Homans DC, Asinger R, Elsperger JK, Erlien D, Sublett E, Mikell F, Bache RJ: Regional function and perfusion at the lateral border of ischemic myocardium. Circulation 71:1038–1047, 1985.
14. Ramanathan K, Bodenheimer MM, Banka VS, Helfant RH: Natural history of contractile abnormalities after acute myocardial infarction in man: severity and response to nitroglycerin as a function of time. Circulation 63:731–738, 1981.
15. Heyndrickx GR, Millard RW, McRitchie RJ, Maroko PR, Vatner SF: Regional myocardial functional and electrophysiological alterations after brief coronary artery occlusion in conscious dogs. J Clin Invest 56:978–985, 1975.
16. Wyatt HL, Meerbaum S: Experimental evaluation of the extent of myocardial dyssynergy and infarct size by two-dimensional echocardiography. Circulation 63:607–614, 1981.
17. Braunwald E, Kloner RA: The stunned myocardium: prolonged post-ischemic ventricular dysfunction. Circulation 66:1146–1149, 1982.
18. Lieberman AN, Weiss JL, Jugdutt BI, Becker LC, Bulkley BH, Garrison JG, Hutchins GM, Kallman CA, Weisfeldt ML: Two-dimensional echocardiography

and infarct size: relationship of regional wall motion and thickening to the extent of myocardial infarction in the dog. Circulation 63:739–746, 1981.

19. Neimeninen M, Parisi AF, O'Boyle JE, Folland ED, Khuri S, Kloner RA: Serial evaluation of myocardial thickening and thinning in acute experimental infarction: identification and quantification using two-dimensional echocardiography. Circulation 66:174–180, 1982.

20. Heger JJ, Weyman AE, Wann LS, Dillon JC, Feigenbaum H: Cross-sectional echocardiography in acute myocardial infarction: detection and localization of regional left ventricular asynergy. Circulation 60:531–538, 1979.

21. Corya BC, Phillips JF, Black MJ, Weyman AE, Rasmussen S: Prevalence of regional left ventricular dysfunction in patients with coronary artery disease. Chest 79:631–637, 1981.

22. Vieweg WVR, Alpert JS, Johnson AD, Dennish GW, Nelson DP, Warren SE, Hagan AD: Distribution and severity of left ventricular wall motion abnormalities according to age and coronary arterial pattern in 500 patients with coronary artery disease and angina pectoris. Am Heart J 99:707–713, 1980.

23. Tomoiki H, Franklin D, Ross J Jr: Detection of myocardial ischemia by regional dysfunction during and after rapid pacing in conscious dogs. Circulation 58:48–56, 1978.

24. Tomoiki H, Franklin D, McKown D, Kemper WS, Guberek M, Ross J Jr: Regional myocardial dysfunction and hemodynamic abnormalities during strenuous exercise in dogs with limited coronary flow. Circ Res 42:487–496, 1978.

25. Smith JS, Cahalan MK, Benefiel DJ, Byrd BF, Lurz FW, Shapiro WA, Roizen MF, Bouchard A, Schiller NB: Intraoperative detection of myocardial ischemia in high risk patients: electrocardiography versus two-dimensional transesophageal echocardiography. Circulation 75:1015–1021, 1985.

26. Clements FM, Hill R, Kisslo J, Orchard R: How easily can we learn to recognize regional wall motion abnormalities with 2-D transesophageal echocardiography? In: Proc Soc Cardiovasc Anesthesiol 7th Annual Meeting, Montreal, May 1986.

27. Burggraf GW, Craige E: Echocardiographic studies of left ventricular wall motion and dimensions after valvular heart surgery. Am J Cardiol 35:473–480, 1975.

28. Miller HC, Gibson DG, Stephens JD: Role of echocardiography and phonocardiography in diagnosis of mitral paraprosthetic regurgitation with Starr-Edwards prostheses. Br Heart J 35:1217–1225, 1973.

29. Vignola PA, Boucher CA, Curfman GD, Walker HJ, Shea WH, Dinsmore RE, Pohost GM: Abnormal interventricular septal motion following cardiac surgery: clinical, surgical, echocardiographic and radionuclide correlates. Am Heart J 97:27–34, 1979.

30. Righetti A, Crawford MH, O'Rourke RA, Schelbert H, Daily PO, Ross J: Interventricular septal motion and left ventricular function after coronary artery bypass surgery. Am J Cardiol 39:372–377, 1977.

31. Force T, Bloomfield P, O'Boyle JE, Khuri SF, Josa M, Parisi AF: Quantitative two-dimensional echocardiographic analysis of regional wall motion in patients with perioperative myocardial infarction. Circulation 70:233–241, 1984.

32. Theroux P, Franklin D, Ross J, Kemper WS: Regional myocardial function during acute coronary artery occlusion and its modification by pharmacologic agents in the dog. Circ Res 35:896–908, 1974.

33. Dubroff JM, Clark MB, Wong CYH, Spotnitz AJ, Collins RH, Spotnitz HM: Left ventricular ejection fraction during cardiac surgery: a two-dimensional echocardiographic study. Circulation 68:95–103, 1983.

34. Roizen MF, Beaupre PN, Alpert RA, Kremer P, Cahalan MK, Schiller N, Sohn YJ, Cronelly R, Lurz FW, Ehrenfeld WK, Stoney RJ: Monitoring with two-dimensional transesophageal echocardiography: comparison of myocardial function in patients undergoing supraceliac, suprarenal–infraceliac, or infrarenal aortic occlusion. J Vasc Surg 1:300–303, 1984.

35. Reichek N, Wilson J, St. John Sutton M, Plappert TA, Goldberg S, Hirshfeld JW: Noninvasive determination of left ventricular end-systolic stress: validation of the method and initial application. Circulation 65:99–108, 1982.

36. Seward JB, Tajik AJ, Spangler JG, Ritter DG: Echocardiographic contrast studies: initial experience. Mayo Clin Proc 50:163–192, 1975.

37. Butler BD, Hills BA: The lung as a filter for microbubbles. J Appl Physiol 47:537–543, 1979.

38. Eguaras MG, Pasalodos J, Gonzalez V, Montero A, Garia MA, Moriones I, Granados J, Valles F, Concha M: Intraoperative two-dimensional echocardiography: evaluation of the presence and severity of aortic and mitral regurgitation during cardiac operations. J Cardiovasc Thorac Surg 89:573–579, 1985.

39. Rodigas PC, Meyer FJ, Haasler GB, Dubroff JM, Spotnitz HM: Intraoperative 2-dimensional echocardiography: ejection of microbubbles from the left ventricle after cardiac surgery. Am J Cardiol 50:1130–1132, 1982.

40. Topol EJ, Humphrey LS, Borkon AM, Baumgartner WA, Dorsey DL, Reitz BA, Weiss JL: Value of intraoperative left ventricular microbubbles detected by transesophageal 2-dimensional echocardiography in predicting neurologic outcome after cardiac operations. Am J Cardiol 56:773–775, 1985.

41. Cucchiara RF, Nugent M, Seward JB, Messick JM: Air embolism in upright neurosurgical patients: detection and localization by two-dimensional transesophageal echocardiography. Anesthesiology 60:353–355, 1984.

42. Henriksen L: Evidence suggestive of diffuse brain damage following cardiac operations. Lancet 1:816–820, 1984.

43. Aberg T, Rouquist G, Tyden H, Brunkvist S, Hultman J, Bergstrom K, Lilja A: Adverse effects on the brain in cardiac operations as assessed by biochemical, psychometric and radiologic methods. J Cardiovasc Thorac Surg 87:99–105, 1984.

44. Lieppe W, Scallion R, Behar VS, Kisslo JA: Two-dimensional echocardiography findings in atrial septal defect. Circulation 56:447–456, 1977.

45. Hanrath P, Schluter M, Langenstein BA, Polster J, Engel S, Kremer P, Krebber H: Detection of ostium secundum atrial septal defects by transesophageal cross-sectional echocardiography. Br Heart J 49:350–358, 1983.

46. Reifart N, Strohm WD, Classen M: Detection of atrial and ventricular septal defects by transesophageal two-dimensional echocardiography with a mechanical sectorscanner. Scand J Gastroenterol [Suppl 94] 19:101–106, 1984.

47. Ezekowitz MD, Smith EO, Rankin R, Harrison LH, Krous HF: Left atrial mass: diagnostic value of transesophageal 2-dimensional echocardiography and indium-111 platelet scintigraphy. Am J Cardiol 51:1563–1564, 1983.

48. Thier W, Schluter M, Krebber H, Polonius M, Kloppel G, Becker K, Hanrath P: Cysts in left atrial myxomas identified by transesophageal cross-sectional echocardiography. Am J Cardiol 51:1793–1795, 1983.

49. Schlüter M, Langenstein BA, Thier W, Schmiegel W, Krebber H, Kalmer P, Hanrath P: Transesophageal two-dimensional echocardiography in the diagnosis of cor triatriatum in the adult. J Am Coll Cardiol 2:1011–1015, 1983.

50. Schlüter M, Kremer P, Hanrath P: Transesophageal 2D echocardiographic feature of flail mitral leaflet due to ruptured chordae tendineae. Am Heart J 108:609–610, 1984.

51. Schlüter MS, Langenstein BA, Hanrath P, Kremer P, Bleifeld W: Assessment of transesophageal pulsed Doppler echocardiography in the detection of mitral regurgitation. Circulation 66:784–789, 1982.
52. Borner N, Erbel R, Braun B, Henkel B, Meyer J, Rumpelt J: Diagnosis of aortic dissection by transesophageal echocardiography. Am J Cardiol 54:1157–1158, 1984.

5. QUANTITATIVE ANALYSIS OF 2D ECHOCARDIOGRAPHIC IMAGES

Two-dimensional cardiac imaging provides an enormous amount of information that can be used to derive quantitative information about cardiac function. A videotape recording is made at a rate of 30 frames per second, so that, for a heart beating at a rate of 60 times per minute, one cardiac cycle amounts to 30 frames of video information. On each video stop-frame, the myocardium is defined by two lines: the epicardium and the endocardium. Therefore, at each stage of the cardiac cycle, two things can be identified: the size of the cavity contained by the endocardium and the thickness of the myocardial wall. We can compare the differences between diastole and systole, and thus estimate how much blood has been ejected or measure how much wall thickening has occurred, but this is information about regional function, derived from a single two-dimensional view of the heart. Global function can be assessed only by considering several views of the left ventricle with echocardiography, unless one can select a view that is fairly representative of global function. It is the echocardiographer who can make the first mistake, therefore, by his selection of an inappropriate 2D view, but having decided upon which part of the left ventricle should be examined, a videotape recording is then made, spanning several cardiac cycles. Although it may be necessary to examine a whole cardiac cycle frame by frame for some analyses, generally it will be enough to examine only those frames taken at end-diastole and end-systole. The identification of these is sometimes done merely by inspection to find the largest and the smallest chamber size, but should more properly be done by gating the image to the ECG. It is sometimes disappointing to find that the quality of the image appears considerably worse as a stop-frame than it did in real time. This is when image recording technique emerges as a fine art. The epicardial and endocardial borders must appear as clearly as possible so that they can be accurately drawn. Missing parts or thickened blurred borders obviously introduce errors in tracing. A number of methods have been devised to trace borders, ranging from the crude method of placing a piece of tracing paper directly on the videoscreen and tracing with a wax pen to the use of a light pen and a graphics tablet. It is certainly preferable to use a light pen, tracing the border directly on the image, since this removes errors due to parallax.

The traced epicardial and endocardial borders are used to measure areas and circumferences for systole and diastole, commonly abbreviated as follows:

EDA = end-diastolic area
ESA = end-systolic area
EDCF = end-diastolic circumference
ESCF = end-systolic circumference

For the various calculations required to measure global and regional function, the traced borders are entered into a digital computer. Various software programs are available for processing the information. The traced borders are converted into pairs of x–y coordinates for digitization, and then a number of parameters can be selected, but it is essential to understand that every calculation stems from a derivation of the digitized outline and so all calculated parameters are only as good as the echocardiographic judgment of how to digitize epi- and endocardial borders. Even a single two-dimensional image contains an enormous amount of digital information. Analysis of a single heartbeat involving 30 frames may exceed the memory capacity of a computer.

In this chapter, some of the pitfalls encountered in quantitative analysis will be examined in detail. The essential prerequisite to understanding such analysis is the understanding of normal left ventricular contraction.

NORMAL LEFT VENTRICULAR CONTRACTION

As recently as 1967 Herman and coworkers [1] defined the normal pattern of left ventricular contraction as a uniform, almost concentric inward motion of all points along the ventricular endocardial surface during systole. Most of the early studies characterizing left ventricular (LV) motion were therefore based on models assuming myocardial fiber structure consistent with uniform contraction. Greenbaum and others [2] showed that myocardial fiber structure is quite complex and that models assuming uniform wall motion are invalid for study of either normal or abnormal ventricles.

Heterogeneous LV wall dynamics have been described with cineangiography and M-mode echocardiography [3–5]. Haendchen and coworkers [6] used transthoracic 2D echocardiography to map regional patterns of contraction in both the canine ventricle and human normal left ventricle: 50 dogs anesthetized with morphine and pentobarbital were studied, of which ten were studied prior to the induction of anesthesia; 32 normal awake human subjects were also studied. Several short-axis views of the LV from the base to the apex were examined.

The mitral valve level was a short-axis view with which both valvular leaflets could be well seen: the high-papillary muscle level included the subvalvular structures, the midpapillary muscle level transected the body of the papillary muscles, and the low-papillary muscle level included the bases of the muscles. A low LV level below the papillary muscles and an apical level with the smallest identifiable luminal area were also examined. Each short-axis view was subdivided into eight segments and these segments were pooled into regions designated as anterior, posterior, septal, and lateral. The septum was considered also in three sections: anterior, middle, and posterior. Wall motion analysis was accomplished by manual tracing of the endocardial and epicardial borders from end-diastolic and end-systolic video stop-frames.

In selecting beats for quantitative analysis, it is important to select beats that are preceded by a sinus beat since a preceding extrasystolic contraction may cause enhanced contractility in the analyzed cardiac cycle. The identification of end-diastole on a stop-frame is done preferably with ECG gating using the peak of the R wave, although it is possible to identify the frame showing the largest cross-sectional area, or it may be defined by the phonocardiographic second heart sound. As with Haendchen's study, most investigators have used end-systolic and end-diastolic frames only; however, it should be noted that

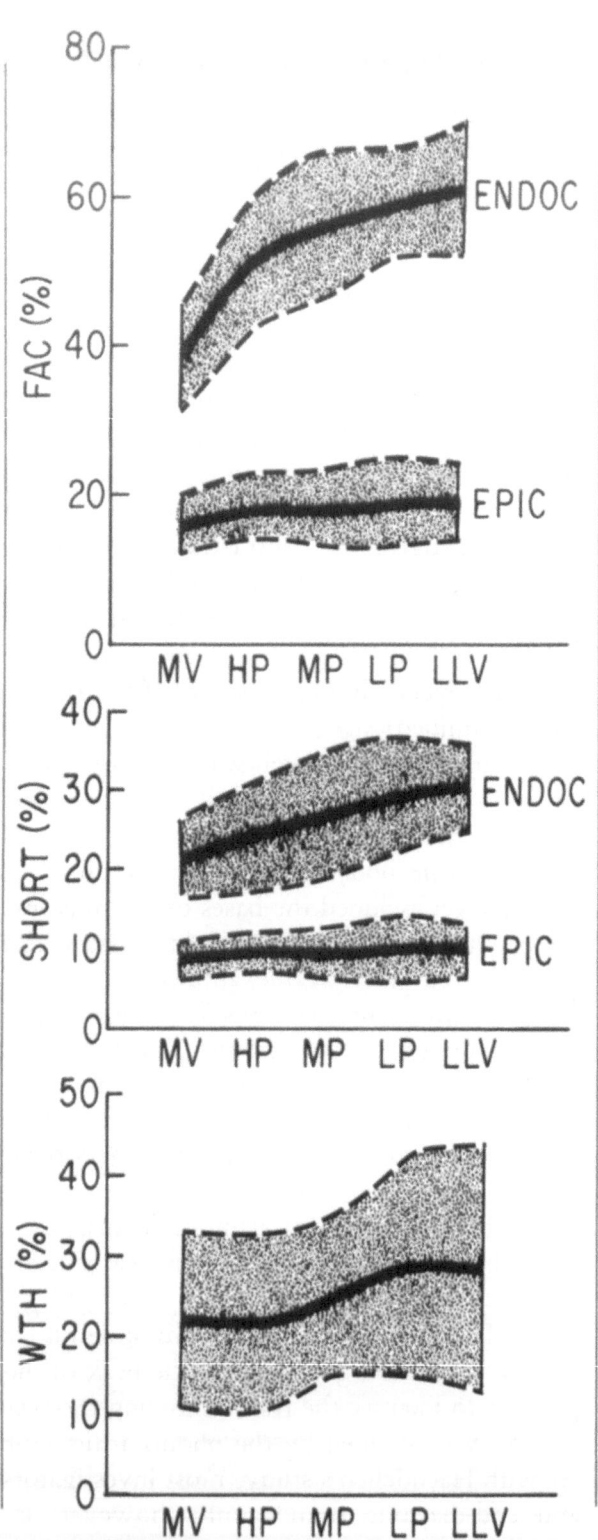

segmental wall motion abnormalities may occur early in systole and can be missed if frame-by-frame analysis through systole is not done. At least some of the commercially available analysis systems incorporate an automated edge detection and tracking program, thus providing the opportunity of frame-by-frame analysis throughout the cardiac cycle. From his data, Haendchen derived three indices of contractile function: systolic fractional area change (of the LV cavity in the short-axis view), wall thickening, and circumferential fiber shortening. Fractional area change (FAC) measures the extent of area change during systole relative to the end-diastolic area; systolic wall thickening (SWTh) measures the change in wall thickness from diastole to systole; circumferential fiber shortening Cfs measures the segmental perimeter shortening relative to the end-diastolic perimeter. FAC and Cfs were derived for both endocardium and epicardium. Because of the more circumferentially oriented fibers in the midwall, shortening was also calculated as the mean value between endo- and epicardial shortening. Haendchen's study showed that, in both the canine and human heart, contraction increases progressively from the base to the apex of the left ventricle. For example, the amplitude of endocardial motion, expressed as the systolic fractional area change, was approximately 40% near the base and 60% near the apex. Although the relative contraction is greatest at the apex, the greatest contribution to stroke volume occurs with area change at the base. Although endocardial FAC, Cfs, and SWTh increased in the direction of the apex, epicardial FAC and Cfs were relatively uniform along the entire left ventricle (figure 5-1).

Kong and coworkers [3], Liedke and others [4], and Leighton and coworkers [7] reported similar findings in humans by using cineventriculography. A good explanation for the base-to-apex variation has not been found. Le Winter and his coworkers [8] postulated that the greater apical shortening might be associated with longer sarcomeres at the LV apex. The thicker layer of circumferentially oriented fibers at the LV base reported by Greenbaum and coworkers [2] could also been responsible for the lesser degree of shortening and thickening at

Figure 5-1. Variations in sectional function from the base to the apex of the left ventricle of 14 normal humans. Results are presented as the mean (solid line) ± 2 SD. MV = mitral valve level, HP = high-papillary muscle level, MP = midpapillary muscle level, LP = low-papillary muscle level, and LLV = low left ventricular level. Reproduced with permission from Haendchen et al. [6].

this level. At the papillary muscle level, there is more inward endo-cardial motion, possibly reflecting a decrease in the circumferentially oriented fibers and an increase in the longitudinally oriented fibers. Marcus and others [9] demonstrated a large myocardial blood flow to the apex to account for an increase in contraction.

The LV exhibits regional variations in endocardial motion and wall thickening around its circumference as well as an intersegmental variation in end-diastolic wall thickness and differences in midwall shortening (figure 5-2). Klausner and coworkers [10] used cineven-triculography to measure segmental wall motion throughout systole and diastole in 32 subjects catheterized for chest pain and found to have normal cardiac function with no significant coronary artery disease. This study indicated that there is heterogeneity of both extent and velocity of wall motion in the normal ventricle and that time-normalized diastolic motion is usually not a mirror image of time-normalized systolic motion in the same segments. Early diastolic relaxation of the anterior wall was found to be consistent with normal diastolic motion [11–13] and events in late diastole are associated with different responses of various regions in the ventricle. Atrial con-traction causes rapid expansion of the anterior wall and apex, while the inferior wall does not change its motion. This variability partly relates to the sequence of electrical activation in the ventricle. Similarly, septal motion is affected by conduction abnormalities since it contains a major part of the conduction system. The ventricular septum is further subject to forces from both the right and left ven-tricles so there are a number of factors that affect its contraction and overall direction of movement.

The interventricular septum comprises about 40% of the LV circumference in the short-axis view, and is made up of muscular and membranous parts. The basal membranous part that lies adjacent to the aortic outflow tract and mitral valve annulus does not contract as the lower muscular portion does. In a normal heart, a short-axis view of the left ventricle at the level of the mitral annulus or immediately below displays anterior movement of the septum, i.e., the septum moves outward from the left ventricle during systole, when the remaining walls of the ventricle contract inward. This paradoxical movement may be misinterpreted as a pathologic dyskinesia. Normally, with systole, the muscular septum thickens by greater than 30% of its diastolic thickness. Paradoxical septal motion is seen in conditions of right ventricular overload that may occur with several conditions, e.g., atrial septal defect, anomalous pulmonary venous drainage, tricuspid insufficiency, and pulmonary hypertension. The effects of right and left bundle branch block on septal motion have also been described [14–18]. With right bundle branch block, the septum moves normally; however, with left bundle branch block, there is generally paradoxical anterior movement of the septum that may be confused with infarction. Right ventricular pacing has also been reported to cause paradoxical septal motion.

SYNCHRONY AND ASYNCHRONY

The normal sequence of electrical activation of the left ventricle can be expected to cause some asynchrony in contraction patterns. Further asynchrony might be expected with the abnormal propagation of the electrical impulse that is prone to occur in and around ischemic tissue. Holman and coworkers [19] studied regional myocardial asynchrony with ECG-gated radionuclide ventriculography in normal subjects, in patients with coronary artery disease but without wall motion abnormalities, and in patients with asynergy during contrast ventriculography. Regional ejection fraction at one-third systole was 0.32 ± 0.02 (mean $\pm$ SEM) in the normals, 0.22 ± 0.01 in patients with coronary artery disease but no asynergy, and 0.12 ± 0.01 in patients with contrast-induced asynergy. In this latter group, severe forms of regional asynchrony appeared in both early systole and early diastole. There appeared from this study to be progressively more regional asynchrony in patients with more severe coronary artery disease. These changes in ejection patterns were qualitatively different from asynchrony seen in normal ventricles; abnormal regions were not delayed as much in the onset of ejection as in the completion of ejection. The degree of ejection of abnormal segments was typically less than that of normal segments early in systole, although by the end of systole many of the abnormal segments were able to achieve normal peak ejection fractions. This relates to the high intraventricular pressures early in systole with the correspondingly high wall stress. Myocardial regions perfused by stenotic vessels have limited functional reserve and their degree of shortening is determined by the relative afterload. Thus, one may expect compromised LV regions to delay active shortening until wall stress has begun to decrease later in systole. With increasingly severe coronary disease, contraction abnormalities appear in early diastole; regional wall contraction may be delayed to the extent that maximum contraction in abnormal segments is occurring during isovolumetric relaxation of the re-

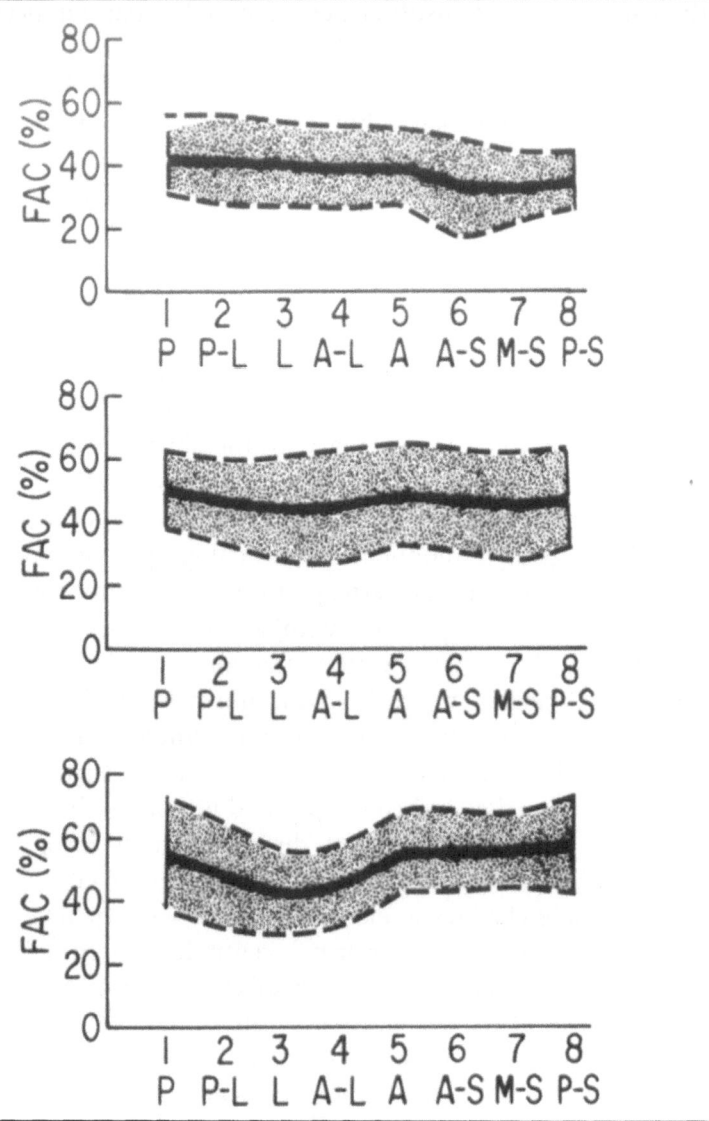

Figure 5-2.

mainder of the ventricle. Concomitantly, early systolic wall motion abnormalites become more severe, with the development of early systolic paradox, or bulging, in the abnormal segment. Thus, the delay in contraction of an ischemic segment may cause an early systolic paradox that is later reversed in early diastole. For these reasons, measurement of end-systolic ventricular contraction alone may sometimes fail to identify normally and abnormally contracting segments.

Paradoxical motion of the interventricular septum has been a par-

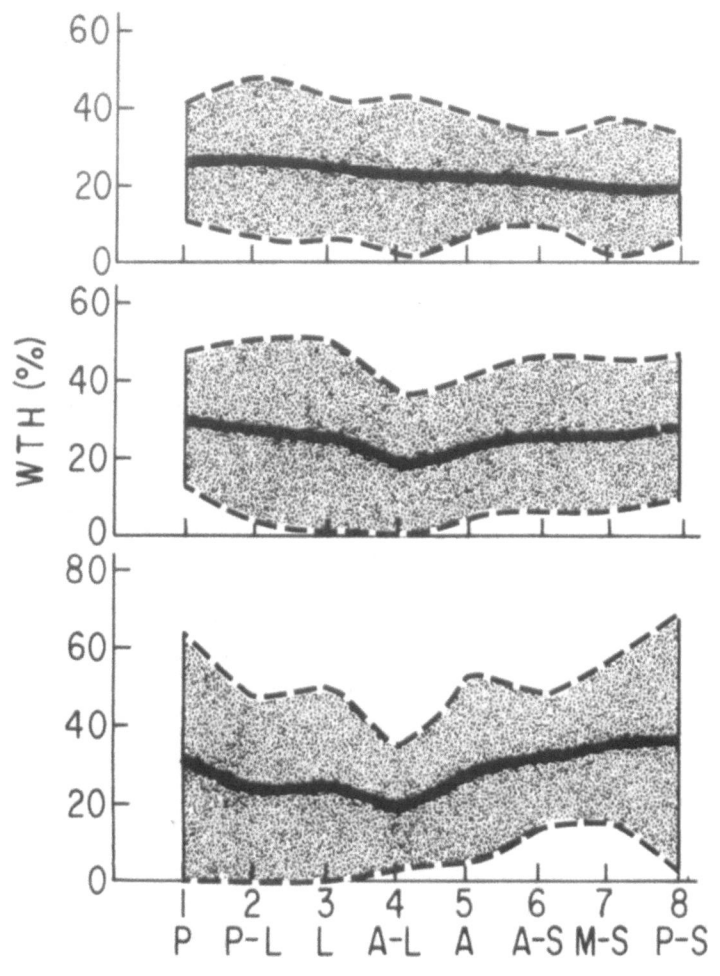

Figure 5-2. Regional differences in FAC (left panel) and WTh (right panel) in normal humans. Differences have been illustrated at mitral valve level (top), midpapillary muscle level (middle), and low left ventricular level (bottom). P = posterior, L = lateral, A = anterior, S = septal, and M = mid. Reproduced with permission from Haendchen et al. [6].

ticularly common feature of patients with coronary artery disease since 75% of its blood supply is derived from the left anterior descending coronary artery [20]. In addition to paradoxical movement of the entire septum, there is also usually reduced systolic septal thickening with stenosis of the left anterior descending coronary artery, and with septal infarction there may be systolic septal thinning. Patients with idiopathic hypertrophic subaortic stenosis may also exhibit reduced systolic thickening of the septum. With this knowledge of the asymmetry of shape and asynchrony of contraction that may characterize the left ventricle, the pitfalls encountered in calculations of global ventricular function must be obvious.

QUANTITATIVE ASSESSMENT OF LEFT VENTRICULAR VOLUME

In order to calculate the volume of a chamber such as the left ventricle, it must first be represented as a mathematical model with dimensions that can be derived from biplane or multiplane data; such models have been used primarily in conjunction with cineangiographic images. The various models and the equations used are represented in figure 5-3. The LV cavity is taken to be similar in shape to a bullet or truncated cone and it is clear that the calculation of volume requires a minimum of two views, e.g., a short axis and a long axis.

All investigators who have examined the correlation between cineangiography and echocardiography for the measurement of ventricular volumes have found significantly smaller end-diastolic volumes with echocardiography than with cineangiography (figure 5-4). There are several possible explanations for this difference. The angiographic outline of the left ventricle includes some areas within the trabeculae that are surrounded by contrast during ventriculography. The echocardiographic definition probably includes the trabeculae with the endocardial border because of the finite lateral resolution of the ultrasound beam (figure 5-5) (see chapter 2).

Also shortening of the long axis due to a failure to image through the apex of the left ventricle or imaging a short-axis plane below the level of maximum cross-sectional area could result in smaller calculated volumes by echocardiography. It should be noted as well that studies comparing volume measurements by echocardiography and cineangiography are comparing measurements that are not collected simultaneously; differences in preload and contractility may account for some disparity in results. Further, it is well known that angiographic contrast medium may depress contractility, although this is not felt to be significant if the images analyzed are recorded within the first three or four beats after contrast injection. Schnittger and co-workers [21] found that end-diastolic LV volume by 2D echocardiography was consistently 20% less than that calculated angiographically in a study of 36 patients with normal and abnormal wall motion. The volume measurements by the two methods correlated well, however ($r > 0.87$). The 20% discrepancy in volume determinations was an

Algorithm	Formula	Geometric model
Simpson's rule I	$V = \dfrac{L}{4}\left[Am + \dfrac{Am + Ap_1}{2} + \dfrac{Ap_1 + Ap_2}{2} + 1/3\ Ap_2 \right]$	
Simpson's rule II	$V = (Amv + Ap_1)\dfrac{L}{3} + \dfrac{Ap_2}{2}\dfrac{L}{3} + \dfrac{\pi}{6}\left(\dfrac{L}{3}\right)^3$	
Hemisphere cylinder (MV)	$V = 5/6\ AL\ (MV)$	
Hemisphere cylinder (PM)	$V = 5/6\ AL\ (PM)$	
Ellipsoid single plane Four-chamber view	$V = 0.85\ A^2/L$	
Ellipsoid single plane Two-chamber view	$V = 0.85\ A^2/L$	
Ellipsoid biplane (MV) Area-length	$V = \pi/6\ L\ D_1\ D_2 (MV)$	
Ellipsoid biplane (PM) Area-length	$V = \pi/6\ L\ D_1\ D_2 (PM)$	

Figure 5-3. Selection of mathematical models used to calculate left ventricular volume.

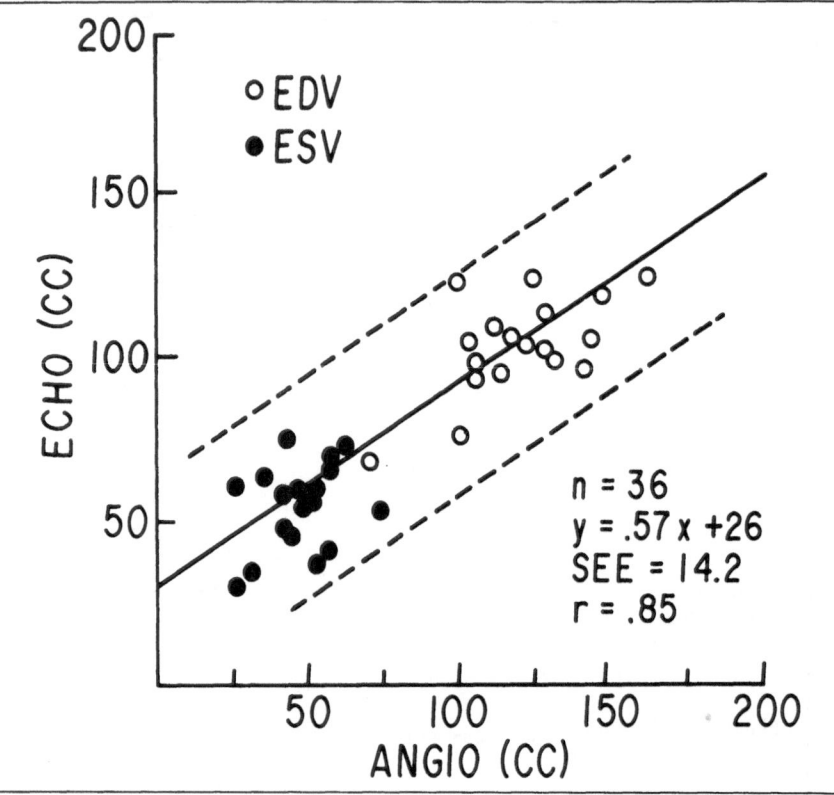

Figure 5-4. End-diastolic (open circles) and end-systolic (closed circles) volumes are plotted for 18 patients whose LV volumes were measured by 2D echocardiography and by cineangiography. Least-squares linear regression yielded $r = 0.85$ and a standard error of the estimate of 14.2 cc; 95% confidence limits are represented by the two dotted lines. Reproduced with permission form Schnittger et al. [21].

improvement over the 30%–40% differences found in many other studies. The suggested reasons for this improvement underscore the importance of several technical details pertaining to the derivation of quantitative information from video data; the investigators in Schnittger's study used a sector scanner incorporating dynamic focusing capability and other features that generated a sharper video image more conducive to accurate tracing; the images were recorded directly onto video disk, without suffering the image degradation inherent in other analyses using videotape; finally, the images were drawn with a light-pen system rather than with a wax pen and tracing paper placed over the image on the screen, as some systems require. In summary, the estimation of ventricular volume is only as good as the images used in the calculation; it must be recognized that in the

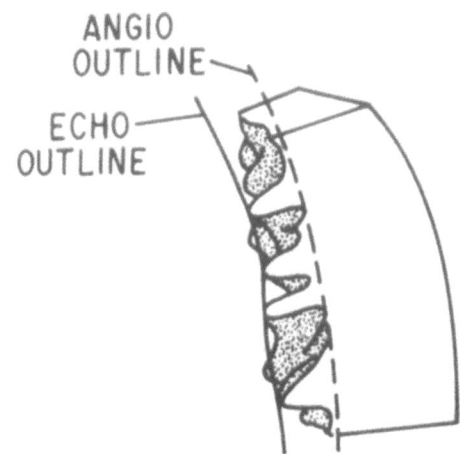

ANGIO
OUTLINE

ECHO
OUTLINE

Figure 5-5. The angiographic outline of the ventricle includes the area of the columnae carneae, since they are surrounded by dye. The echocardiographic outline probably represents the apices of the columnae. Reproduced with permission from Schnittger et al. [21].

presence of regional wall motion abnormalities, especially gross abnormalities such as those created by a ventricular aneurysm, the calculated volume is invalidated. For such asymmetrically contracting ventricles it becomes necessary to use formulas that include multiple sectional views through the ventricle such as Simpson's rule, which employs several short-axis cross-sectional views (figure 5-3). Presently available esophageal transducers emit a fan-shaped ultrasound beam in a single plane only. Therefore, the transducer must be moved in order to obtain more than one view. However, an orthogonal transducer system may become available with which long- and short-axis views are obtained at the same time by directing two ultrasound beams simultaneously, in different planes. This would facilitate the measurement of volume. Until then, the transesophageal echocardiographer is committed to moving the transducer to record enough views for volume calculation, or he can consider a single planar view as representative of ventricular volume, and can derive ejection phase indices from area rather than volume data. It is well established that minor axis shortening is by far the most important factor determining stroke volume. Rankin and coworkers [22] found in chronically instrumented dogs that minor axis shortening accounted for 87% of the stroke volume. Thus, short-axis areas are quite representative of LV volumes.

EJECTION FRACTION AND CIRCUMFERENTIAL SHORTENING

Ejection fraction is taken to refer to that fraction of diastolic volume ejected from the LV during systole, expressed by:

$$EF\ (\%) = \frac{EDV - ESV}{EDV} \times 100$$

where EDV = end-diastolic volume and ESV = end-systolic volume. Similar information can be gained from measuring the LV cavity area in the short-axis plane. This area ejection fraction (AEF), also referred to as a fractional area change (FAC), should provide a good indication of LV ejection. Area ejection fraction or fractional area change in the short-axis is expressed as:

$$AEF\ (\%) = \frac{EDA - ESA}{EDA} \times 100$$

where EDA = end-diastolic area and ESA = end-systolic area. At a midpapillary level, AEF = approximately 50%. Similarly, percent shortening of the endocardial diameter or perimeter, a linear dimension rather than area, can be used to describe ventricular function. For LV diameter, this is expressed by:

$$\%FS = \frac{EDD - ESD}{EDD} \times 100$$

where EDD = end-diastolic endocardial diameter and ESD = end-systolic endocardial diameter. Both AEF and %FS are equivalent to ejection fraction and are pre- and afterload dependent; as with ejection fractions, they become inaccurate in the presence of ventricular wall motion abnormalities.

Endocardial circumference has also been used for derivation of V_{cf}, the velocity of circumferential shortening. There is an abundance of literature supporting V_{cf} as a valuable index of LV performance in infants, children, and adults [23–26]. The added element of time allows for better separation of normal and abnormal LV function than ejection fraction alone. Mean V_{cf} is calculated as:

$$V_{cf} = \frac{EDP - ESP}{EDD \times LVET} \text{ (circumferences/s)}$$

where EDP = end-diastolic endocardial perimeter, ESP = end-systolic endocardial perimeter, and LVET = left ventricular ejection time. Nixon and coworkers [26] studied healthy subjects with a head-down tilt of 5° and during progressively lower-body negative pressures and concluded that V_{cf} is an index of contractility that is largely independent of preload.

QUANTITATION OF LEFT VENTRICULAR MUSCLE MASS AND STRESS

The measurement of LV muscle mass is the accepted standard for identifying the presence of LV hypertrophy. All echocardiographic calculations of muscle mass are based on the assumption that the volume of the myocardium is equal to the total volume contained within the epicardial border of the ventricle minus the volume of the ventricular cavity. Assuming the specific mass of the myocardium, myocardial volume can be converted to mass. In LV mass calculations, the interventricular septum is considered to be a part of the left ventricle.

In dilated ventricles, ventricular wall thickness has to increase proportionally in order to prevent an increase in wall stress. In pressure overload situations, one finds an increase in ventricular mass that appears excessive for the chamber volume; whereas, in volume overload, a constant relationship between LV volume and mass is generally maintained. Thus, the appropriate increase of ventricular muscle mass, or hypertrophy, maintains a normal peak systolic stress even with high peak systolic LV pressures or with substantial ventricular dilation. Echocardiographic images provide a way to measure myocardial mass, wall thickness, and thus stress, since wall stress is represented by:

$$\text{stress} = \frac{\text{pressure} \times \text{radius}}{\text{wall thickness}}$$

Noninvasive determination of wall stress has been evaluated by Quinones and coworkers [27] and by Reichek and others [28]. Stress represents force per unit area of the myocardial wall and measures ventricular load at the specified time in the cardiac cycle. The stress acting along the circumference of the left ventricle at its minor axis is directly related to the intracavitary pressure and to the radius of curvature, and is inversely related to wall thickness. Thus, the increase in myocardial mass with compensatory hypertrophy is indicated by an increase in wall thickness on the echocardiographic image.

End-diastolic stress can be determined by end-diastolic pressure, wall thickness, and radius of the short-axis LV image. During systole, the intracavitary pressure first rises and then falls while wall thickness steadily increases. The net effect of these changes is that wall stress, or afterload, varies with time. Afterload has therefore been described by peak, mean, or end-systolic wall stress.

Quinones and coworkers [27] calculated three indices of LV wall stress, at end-systole, at end-diastole, and as a mean value, using the following equations that lend themselves to use with echocardiographic data:

$$WS_{es} = \frac{\text{systolic arterial pressure} \times \text{radius}}{\text{end-systolic wall thickness}}$$

$$WS_{ed} = \frac{\text{systolic arterial pressure} \times \text{radius}}{\text{end-diastolic wall thickness}}$$

$$\text{mean stress} = \frac{\text{systolic arterial pressure} \times \text{mean radius}}{\text{mean wall thickness}}$$

With these formulas, it appears that peak circumferential wall stress can be accurately estimated noninvasively in a variety of cardiac conditions. Reichek and coworkers [28] developed a method for the noninvasive estimation of wall stress using cuff systolic arterial pressure and M-mode echocardiography. End-systolic LV meridional wall stress is a quantitative index of myocardial afterload that can be plotted against LV end-systolic diameter to give an index of contractility independent of loading conditions. They observed that cuff systolic arterial pressure correlated well with end-systolic LV pressure ($r = 0.89$) and "noninvasive stress" correlated well with "invasive stress" measurements ($r = 0.97$). Other investigators have, approximating the left ventricle to the shape of a thin-walled sphere, found a close relationship between myocardial oxygen consumption ($M\dot{V}O_2$) and peak wall tension; tension equals stress in a wall of zero thickness. Several studies indicate that peak wall stress is a major mechanical index of myocardial oxygen consumption, and the ability to measure it in clinical care would provide an index of myocardial well-being that is not presently available for routine use.

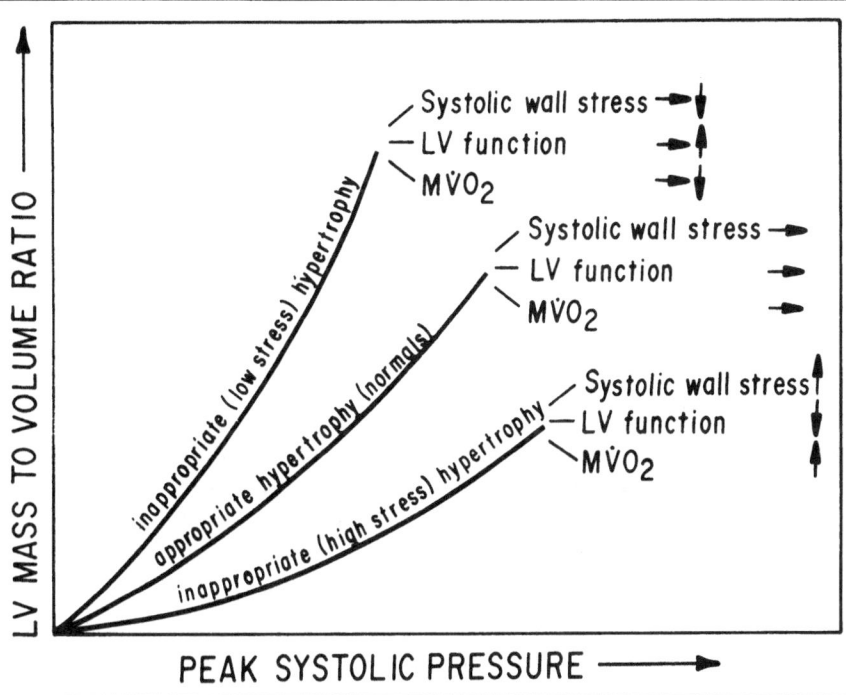

Figure 5-6. Classification of hypertrophic heart disease with regard to the degree or appropriateness of left ventricular hypertrophy. MVO$_2$ = Myocardial oxygen consumption. Reproduced with permission from Strauer [29].

LEFT VENTRICULAR HYPERTROPHY AND WALL STRESS

Strauer [29] found that the relationship of LV hypertrophy to LV cavity size profoundly influenced both LV function and myocardial oxygen consumption (figure 5-6). High-stress hypertrophy, in which there is excessive LV dilation for the amount of LV hypertrophy, was associated with an increase in myocardial oxygen consumption and depressed LV function. Low-stress hypertrophy, however, in which there is a marked increase in LV mass out of proportion to the LV cavity size, was associated with normal or increased LV function and normal or low myocardial oxygen consumption. Appropriate, compensatory hypertrophy was associated with normal oxygen and LV performance.

END-SYSTOLIC INDICES OF VENTRICULAR PERFORMANCE

Since some indices of ventricular performance, like ejection fraction, are dependent on the loading conditions (preload and afterload), there has recently been great interest in end-systolic indices of ventricular performance that are independent of loading conditions. Echocardiography, by providing dimensional data, allows us access to these more precise measures of inotropic state. Suga and Sagawa, using an isolated heart preparation, characterized end-systolic pressure–volume relationships and established the usefulness of this relationship for characterizing myocardial contractility [30–32] (figure 5-7). Many studies have investigated the applications of various end-systolic indices in animal and human subjects. In cardiac muscle fibers studied at the sarcomere level, peak force generated during isosarcometric contraction defines the contractile function of the muscle. Extrapolation of these observations to the study of the intact ventricle involves a number of assumptions; the left ventricle is assumed to have a spherical or ellipsoid shape, and its dimensions are taken from echocardiographic or cineangiographic images (see above).

The ventricular wall is assumed to be uniform in thickness and its mechanical properties homogeneous; excitation of the ventricle is assumed to be instantaneous so that contraction of all parts occurs simultaneously. With these assumptions, contractility can be assessed from the calculated end-systolic force–length relations. The end-systolic force–length relation is approximately linear in cardiac muscle for resting (end-diastolic) sarcomere lengths between 1.2 and 2.1 microns. This range of lengths corresponds to normal LV diastolic volumes. Thus, the relationship between force and length at end-systole is represented by the slope E_{es}, the end-systolic elastance. End-systolic data from echocardiographic dimensions and some approximation of peak systolic LV pressure provide us with two indices of contractility: E_{es} and peak force. If the ventricular wall is damaged by infarction, the validity of these indices is lost; an apparent loss of contractility may reflect absence of contractility in the infarct area, but the remaining myocardium may have enhanced contractility. However, pressure–volume analysis in nonhomogeneous ventricles may still be of value in describing global ventricular function and predicting the interactions of the heart with the peripheral circulation. In normal hearts, pressure–volume analysis has been used to study the effects of drugs on contractility.

CELLULAR DEFINITION OF CONTRACTILITY

Contractility has always been a difficult quantity to measure. Peak systolic force depends on two variables: the concentration of free calcium ions made available to the actin filaments and the affinity of

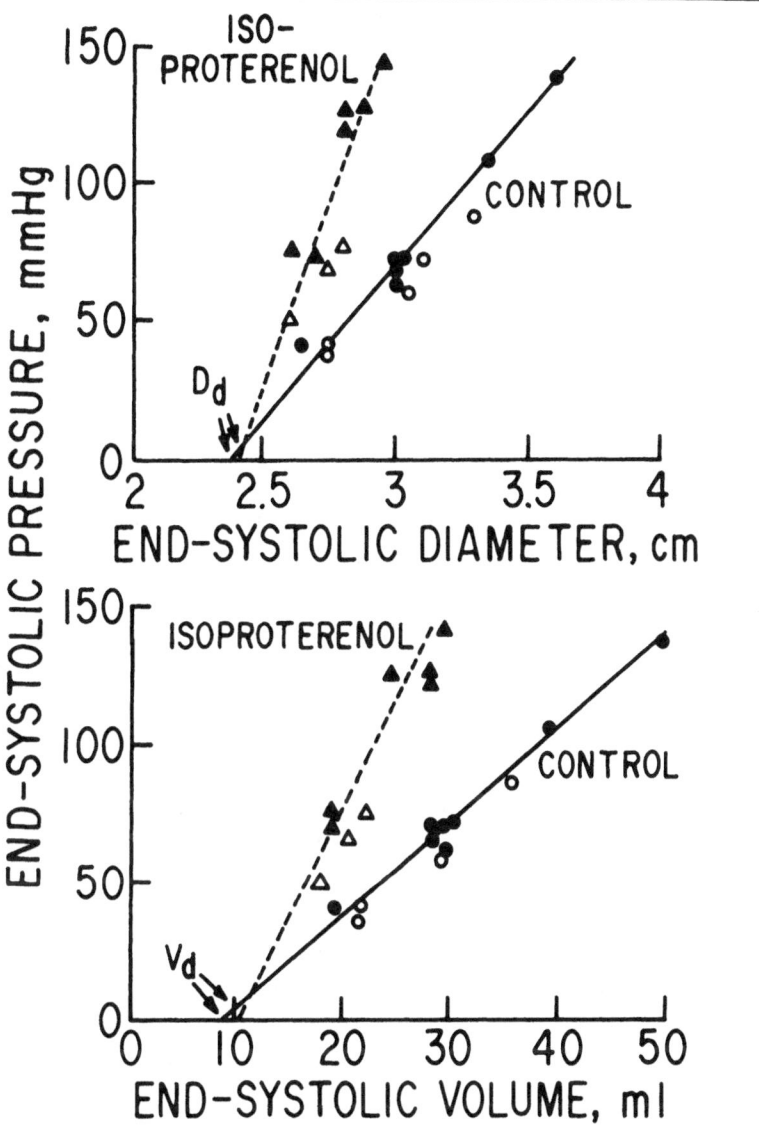

Figure 5-7. Shifts of the end-systolic pressure–diameter and pressure–volume relations with enhancement of the contractile state by intracoronary infusion of isoproterenol. Modified with permission from Sagawa [30].

the troponin–tropomyosin molecules for calcium. This latter variable is related to the degree of phosphorylation of troponin, and the concentration of available calcium is related to the complex calcium flux mechanisms occurring in the cell. The net effect of the calcium fluxes may vary from beat to beat, because of time dependency of outer membrane calcium transport and because of uptake, transport, and release of sarcoplasmic calcium. Several external factors influence these processes, including temperature, ion concentrations, catecholamine levels, and cyclic AMP and cyclic GMP levels. The "inotropic" effects of drugs can be traced back to these biochemical interactions.

DIASTOLIC PRESSURE–VOLUME RELATIONS

Although the observation of systolic contraction is the most impressive feature provided by 2D echocardiography, the behavior of the myocardium during its phase of relaxation, diastole, has proven to be extremely sensitive to ischemia and other abnormalities (figure 5-8). Diastolic pressure–volume relations may therefore generate more attention with the availability of a noninvasive tool for their study. Diastole is characterized by time-varying elastance, which is most obvious during the early phase of LV filling occurring while LV pressure is still falling. Diastolic myofilament interaction is present normally in resting cardiac muscle [33–36] and varies depending on heart rate and inotropic state. Both acute and chronic changes in the diastolic pressure–volume relation may be seen in patients with coronary artery disease. Chronic elevations in LV diastolic pressures with normal volumes have been observed in some patients with coronary artery disease [37, 38], probably due to extensive myocardial fibrosis; Gibson and coworkers [39, 40] identified chronic regional diastolic wall motion abnormalities in similar patients and concluded that this was not necessarily due to ischemia or infarction, but may have been a manifestation of a stable modification or degradation in function seen in areas supplied by diseased coronaries. Deliberately induced ischemia, by pacing, has been observed to increase LV diastolic pressures by several investigators [41–45]. The upward shift in the diastolic pressure–volume relation can be quite dramatic. Mechanisms for this increase in diastolic stiffness may include impaired relaxation, altered diastolic tone, tension prolongation during recovery from hypoxia, and even partial ischemic contracture of some myofibrils within the region supplied by the stenotic artery. As a unifying hypothesis [46], it is possible that the ischemic myocardial cell is confronted with both increased net calcium influx and a decreased rate and quantity of calcium sequestration. Increased intracellular calcium could result from increased inward movement and/or decreased calcium efflux during each cardiac cycle. These alterations in

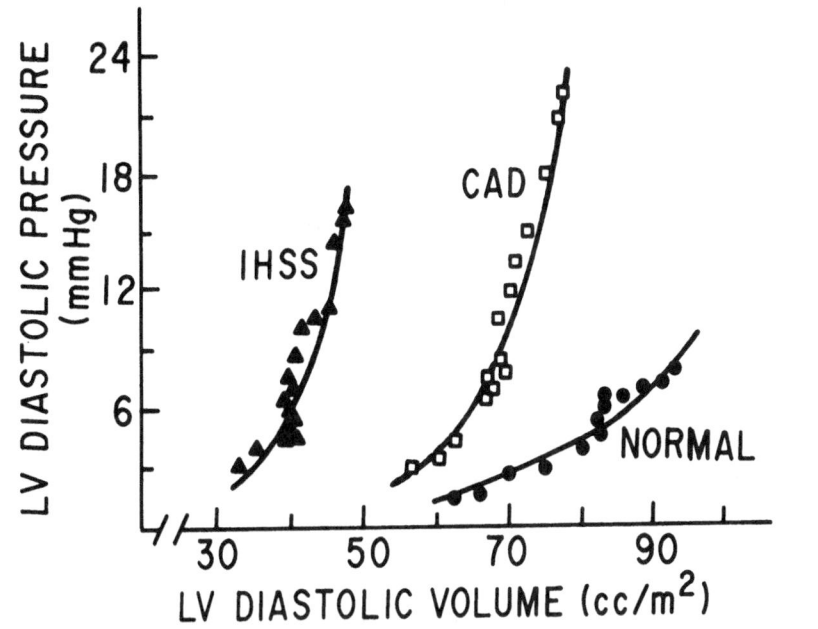

Figure 5-8. Left ventricular pressure–volume data from three subjects: one with hypertrophic cardiomyopathy (IHSS), one with coronary heart disease (CAD), and one with a normal heart. In IHSS, the diastolic pressure–volume curve is displaced to the left of normal, as with CAD. Reproduced with permission from authors and publisher of *Am. J. Cardiol* 38:645, 1976.

calcium flux probably represent a decreased availability of ATP in the sarcoplasmic reticulum.

QUANTITATION OF REGIONAL SYSTOLIC WALL MOTION ABNORMALITIES

The occurrence of regional systolic wall motion abnormalities has proved to be a sensitive and specific marker for ischemia and infarction, the abnormality being potentially reversible if due to ischemia alone. For this reason, and because 2D echocardiography is so well suited to the study of regional wall motion, there has been considerable interest in both the qualitative and quantitative assessment of wall motion, which is already well established in cineangiography for the study of regional differences in myocardial blood flow. Although some investigators have used quantitative techniques [47–52], most still rely on qualitative assessment. With cineangiography, the ventriculogram is used for assessment of wall motion. Opacification of the ventricular cavity with contrast obviously identifies the endocardium only, and provides a silhouette in one or two selected planes. 2D echocardiography however, allows much more flexibility, since it is noninvasive, allows visualization of the entire left ventricle by a combination of views, and most importantly it provides visualization of both endocardium and epicardium. Systolic wall motion abnormalities by 2D echocardiography therefore comprise endocardial movement, circumferential shortening of endocardial and epicardial borders, and systolic wall thickening. Endocardial movement, representing at a global level LV ejection, is expressed regionally as a regional ejection fraction or segmental ejection fraction. For all investigators, the description of regional wall motion has involved, first, the designation of the different 2D views of the left ventricle and, second, the division of each view into a number of segments. There has then remained the question of how to digitize the analog video data and which method of analysis to use. The definition of normal and abnormal regional wall motion has been confounded by these difficulties in making quantitative measurements, since the amplitude of wall motion for various areas of the myocardium has been shown to vary as a function of the method of analysis [52]. Furthermore, the pattern of contraction in the left ventricle is not uniform or concentric, as was previously assumed.

METHODS AND MODELS FOR REGIONAL WALL MOTION ANALYSIS: FIXED AND FLOATING REFERENCE SYSTEMS

In the quantitative analysis of regional wall motion, there are a number of considerations that affect validity. Many investigations have been concerned with the factors that enhance the sensitivity and reproducibility of wall motion analyses. Computerized analyses examine the systolic change in length of chords or radii of the ventricle, or examine systolic area changes of ventricular segments. The number of radii or segments into which the ventricle is divided can be varied, making it difficult to compare results of different studies. For each cardiac cycle, the digital data derived from the video image in systole and diastole must somehow be compared and, in order to do this, the movement of various regions of myocardium must be referenced to some point. There are two major groups of reference systems in common use for this purpose. Fixed reference systems reference the endocardial outlines to some fixed point of reference, either an internal one marked by an anatomic landmark within the heart on the video image, or an external landmark outside the heart. Using such a fixed point of reference, the systolic and diastolic images are superimposed and the distance between the systolic and diastolic borders of each segment is measured by computer. If, during systole, the heart rotates or shifts within the chest cavity, the fixed external reference systems will include this translational or rotational movement as wall motion.

Floating-axis reference systems, however, use a calculated center of mass as the reference point for the video images, superimposing the centers of mass of the end-systolic and end-diastolic images prior to measuring the endocardial excursion with systole. In this way, the floating-axis systems correct for translational movement. The internal anatomic landmarks used to correct for rotational movement may be the papillary muscles or sometimes the insertion point of the right ventricle onto the interventricular septum.

The validity of the different reference methods has been examined by several investigators with transthoracic 2D images, but similar evaluations with transesophageal images have not been reported. Schnittger and coworkers [53] studied 61 subjects with the use of 44 variations of the different reference methods to compare their accuracy in the quantitative analysis of ventricular wall motion. Parasternal short-axis views at the mitral valve and papillary muscle levels were used, in addition to an apical four-chamber view. The broad categories of reference methods employed included a fixed external reference, a floating reference correcting for translation, and a floating reference correcting for both translation and rotation. Initially, the LV wall motion of 20 normal subjects was analyzed and plotted to obtain a 95% confidence interval for each of the 44 methods. Subsequently, the wall motion of an additional ten normal and 31 abnormal subjects was compared with the initial group. This study revealed that the absolute values for LV wall motion varied markedly with different reference methods applied to the same 2D view, and also when the same reference method was applied to different views.

Fixed external reference systems generally resulted in wider normal bands than did floating-axis methods. For each reference method, the band of normal wall motion was wider for a short-axis view at the level of mitral valve than for one at the papillary muscle level. At the mitral valve level, there was approximately 5° of rotation with systole. The fulcrum of torsion seemed to be in the body of the left ventricle at the midpapillary muscle level. Rotation therefore is a negligible problem with a short-axis view at the papillary muscle level, and translational movement was also found to be minimal at this level. Therefore, a fixed reference wall motion analysis method proved to be perfectly satisfactory for the short-axis view at the papillary muscle level, and in fact was superior to the floating reference systems for this view. Sensitivity and specificity for normal wall motion at this level were both 95%, clearly superior to the values obtained with other 2D views. These results compare well with those of Parisi and coworkers [54], who, with slightly different methodology, reported sensitivity at 95%, specificity 89%, and predictive accuracy 92% with a fixed reference analysis of the same LV view (figures 5-9 and 5-10).

DESCRIPTORS OF REGIONAL WALL MOTION

In 2D echocardiography, the systolic movement of the ventricular wall is measured by dividing it into multiple radii or areas. Generally only the endocardial border and the LV cavity contained within it have been considered. However, the same divisions can be applied to the actual ventricular wall to describe regional differences in systolic wall thickening. For a number of reasons, the use of wall thickening rather than endocardial movement alone may be preferable to describe wall motion.

Several investigators have examined the advantages of dividing the ventricular image into radii versus areas, usually considering only the endocardial border. Grube and coworkers [55] found a slight advantage of area over radial methods; Parisi and coworkers [54] reported predictive accuracy to be better with an area method than with a radial method, in conjunction with a fixed reference system. There was no difference between area and radial methods, however, when a floating-axis system was employed. The work of Schnittger and colleagues [53] evaluated the use of varying numbers of image subdivisions and found no difference between area and radial methods with image subdivisions up to 45°; 5°–30° sampling intervals were recommended for either method.

OBSERVER VARIABILITY

With either area or linear radial measurements, different results may be obtained by different observers, and by the same observer examining images at different times.

Moynihan and coworkers [52] studied interobserver variability and found a range of 3.3%–6% for linear measurements and 5.5%–9.7%

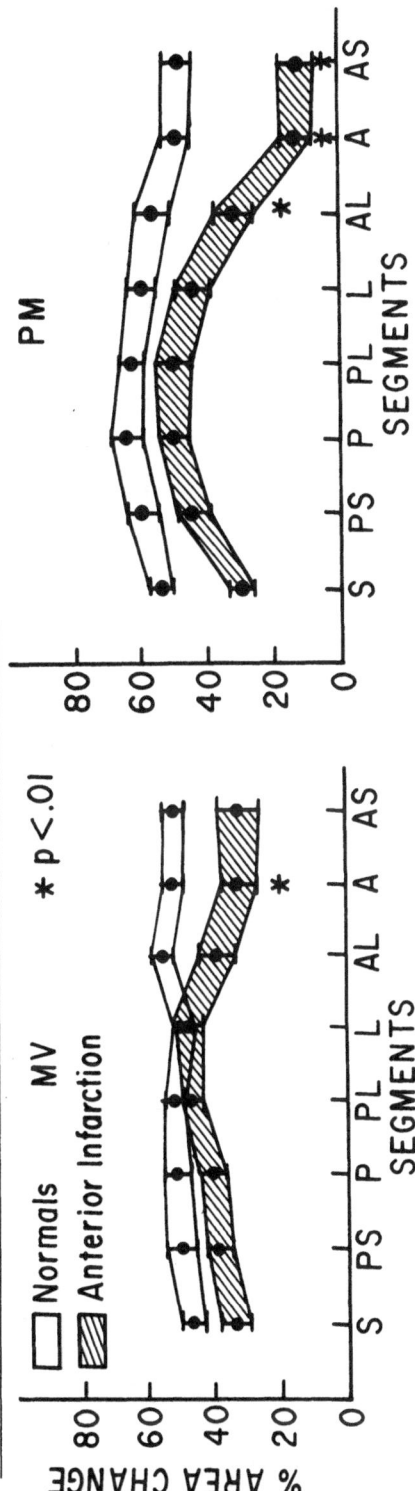

Figure 5-9. Plots of regional contraction (mean ± SEM) as measured by a fixed-axis octant area method in patients with an anterior myocardial infarction and normal volunteers. Data from the mitral valve (MV) level are plotted at the left, and the papillary muscle level data (PM) are plotted at the right. S = septal, PS = posteroseptal, P = posterior, PL = posterolateral, L = lateral, AL = anterolateral, A = anterior, and AS = anteroseptal. Reproduced with permission from Parisi et al. [54].

110

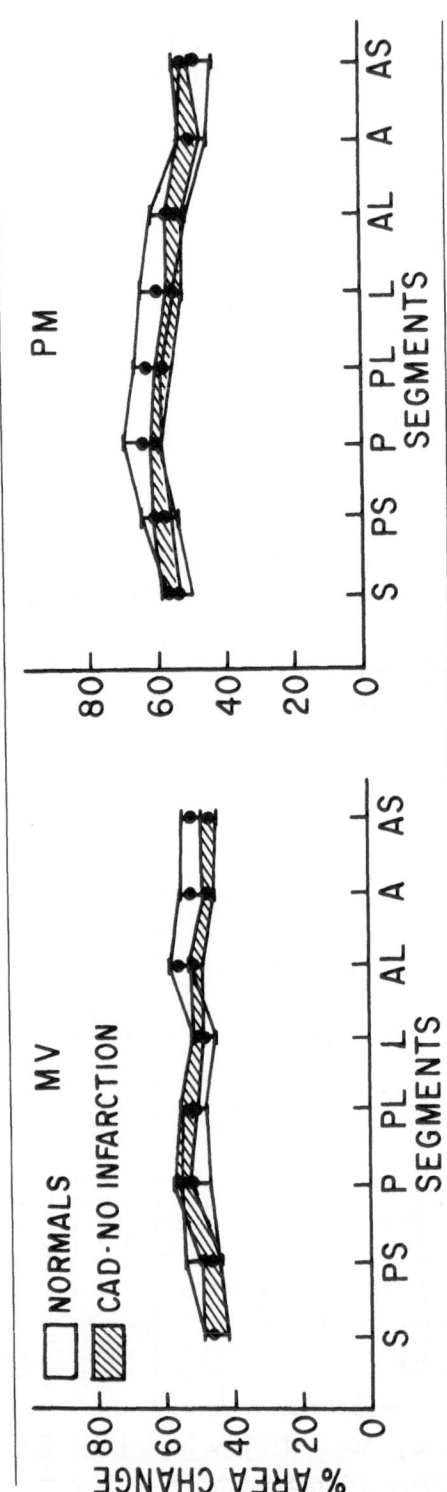

Figure 5-10. Plots of regional contraction (mean ± SEM) for patients with coronary artery disease without infarction, versus normal volunteers. Regional contraction was not significantly different in any region. Format and abbreviations as in figure 5-9. Reproduced with permission from Parisi et al. [54].

for area measurements. This was not affected by the use of fixed versus floating reference systems. Schnittger and coworkers [53] noted that analyses of the same subject on different days occasionally revealed variations of up to 16% for radial methods and 22% for area methods. This day-to-day variability may reflect biologic variability. Pandian and Kerber [56] found that intraobserver variability, with the same observer analyzing the same images at different times, was as high as 20.4% for segmental area change measurements. Haendchen and coworkers [6] found interobserver variability for end-systolic areas to be larger than for end-diastolic areas, reflecting the larger size and better definition of end-diastolic endocardial borders. Interobserver variability for wall thickness measurements, however, was less than 7%. In summary, the use of fixed versus floating-axis, radii versus areas, remains a controversial issue. It appears, however, that the problem of cardiac rotation and translation can be completely circumvented by the consideration of systolic wall thickening rather than endocardial motion alone.

MEASUREMENT OF WALL THICKNESS

The accuracy of wall thickness measurements relies on the accuracy of epicardial and endocardial edge detection. By 2D echocardiography, systolic wall thickening of the human LV free wall varies from 40% to 80% [57–59]. In animals, however, values of 10%–30% are reported [60–62]. Measurements in animals, however, have usually been made with more direct techniques than transthoracic 2D echocardiography, via miniature piezoelectric crystals sutured directly onto the endo- and epicardial surfaces. The discrepancy between the human and animal values for systolic wall thickening has been ascribed to the inclusion of compressed trabeculae carneae in the apparent systolic wall thickness by echocardiography. Feneley and Hickie [63] examined the question of whether echocardiographic techniques overestimate the systolic wall thickness. They studied 18 normal subjects in whom 2D echocardiograms were recorded of the LV short axis, at a midpapillary muscle level. The endocardial and epicardial outlines were traced and planimetered. The leading edge of the echo borders nearest and furthest away from the transducer was followed during tracing, with the lateral echoes being bisected, according to the recommendations of Wyatt and coworkers [64] (see below). End-systolic and end-diastolic myocardial cross-sectional areas (Myo CSA) were calculated as follows:

ES Myo CSA = ESepi CSA − ESendo CSA

ED MYO CSA = EDepi CSA − EDendo CSA

In this study, systolic wall thickening averaged 50%, exceeding the values reported in animal studies. The investigators reasoned that, since myocardial cross-sectional area is a function of wall thickness and wall circumference, overestimation of systolic wall thickening by echocardiography would be expected to involve an overestimation of end-systolic myocardial cross-sectional area relative to end-diastolic cross-sectional area. In fact they found, by linear regression analysis, a close correlation between the two parameters with the slope of the regression line approaching unity (figure 5-11). Their results suggested that there is not a significant overestimation of systolic wall thickening by 2D echocardiographic techniques. Further, work by Pandian and Kerber [56], comparing the measurements obtained by 2D-echocardiography with those derived from implanted piezoelectric crystals, has confirmed the correlation of these two techniques.

ACCURACY IN TRACING BORDERS

Wyatt and coworkers [64] tested several methods in vitro for the accuracy of linear and cross-sectional measurements and in vivo for LV volume reconstruction. They made images with high- and low-gain settings, and traced the myocardial borders with several methods (figure 5-12). The myocardial borders imaged by echocardiography have a thickness defined by the echoes reflected by the myocardial surface. This thickness is magnified with high-gain settings and therefore accurate border tracing becomes more difficult. The leading edge of the border is the edge nearest to the transducer, whereas the trailing edge is that furthest away. For borders lying perpendicular to the ultrasound beam definition is good, but in the lateral field borders tend to be less well defined. Wyatt and coworkers [64] compared the accuracy of tracing borders by the leading–trailing, the trailing–leading, and the leading–leading methods. The first of these requires the observer to trace from the leading edge of the border closest to the transducer to the trailing edge of the more distant border, traversing the middle of the echoes in the lateral field. This method therefore includes most of the width of the entire circumferential border. The trailing–leading method is the reverse of this, excluding almost the entire width of the border and resulting in a smaller circumferential

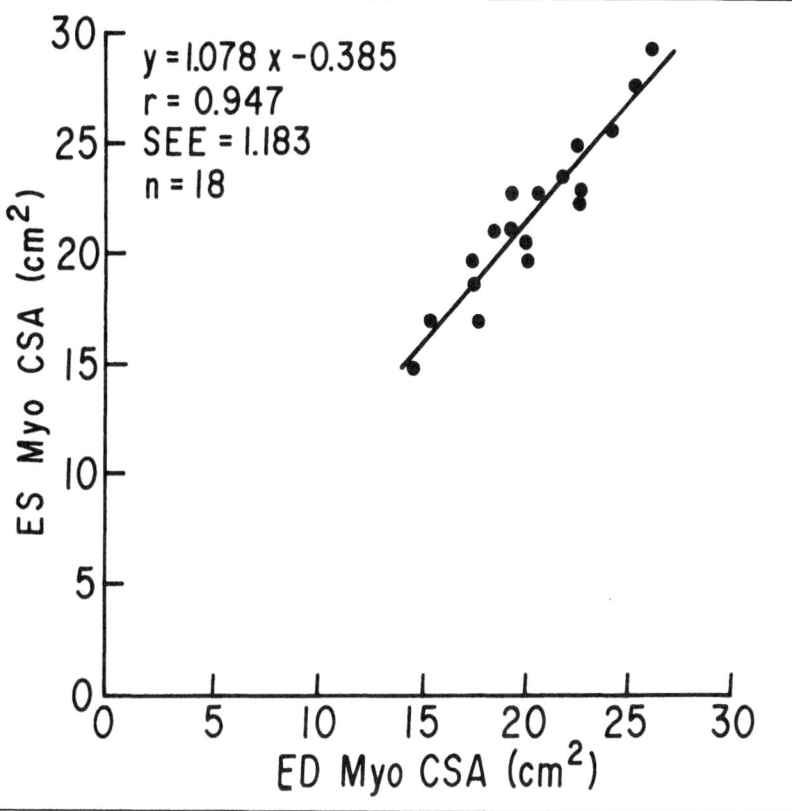

Figure 5-11. Correlation of ES Myo CSA and ED Myo CSA at the midpapillary muscle level of the left ventricle in 18 normal subjects. Reproduced with permission from Feneley and Hickie [63].

measurement. The leading–leading method includes the width of the border nearest the transducer, but excludes the border furthest away.

Regression analysis of the in vitro study comparing 2D echo versus direct measurements yielded excellent correlations for all three methods ($r > 0.985$) with interobserver variability of <3%. Accuracy of the measurements, however, was satisfactory only for the leading–leading method, which had a 3% and 6% error at low- and high-gain, respectively. The other two methods overestimated or underestimated wall thickness substantially. With in vivo comparison of LV volumes by cineangiography and 2D echocardiography, the leading edge method of defining the borders again resulted in the least error. As with endocardial motion, there are important regional differences in systolic wall thickening of the normal human left ventricle [6] with a progressive increase from base to apex. Around the minor axis cir-

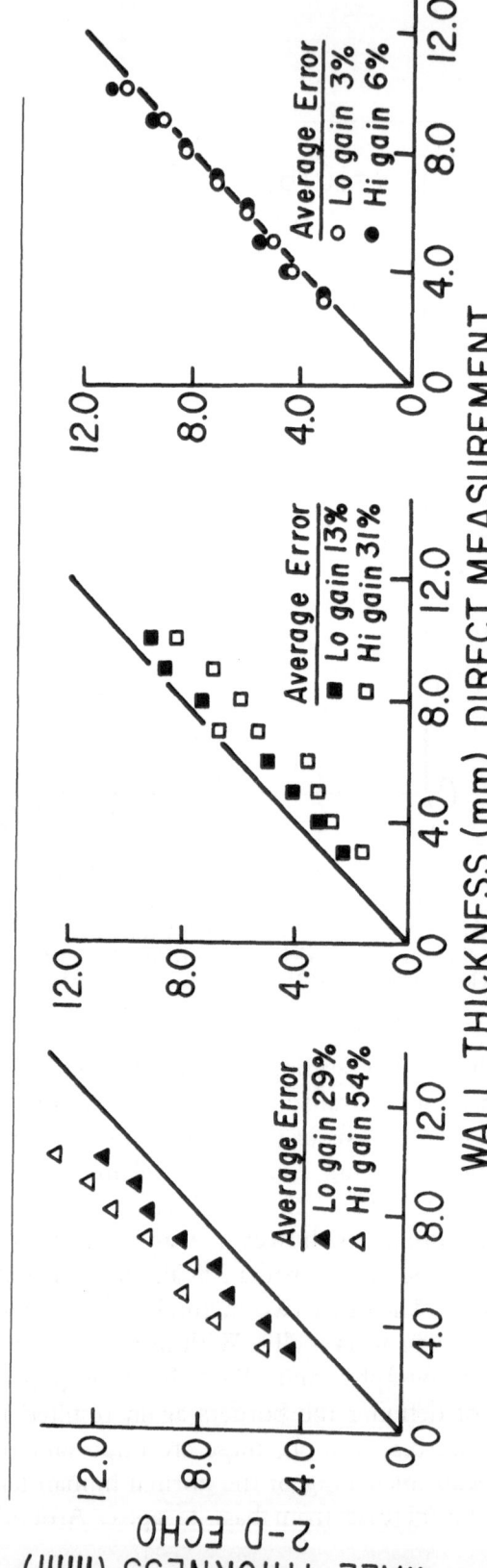

Figure 5-12. Comparison of *in vitro* myocardial thickness measurements, direct (x-axis) versus 2D echocardiography (y-axis) with (left) leading–trailing, (middle) trailing–leading, and (right) leading–leading methods in the presence of low gain or high gain. Reproduced with permission from Wyatt et al. [64].

cumference of the left ventricle, there are also regional differences, with posterior segments showing apparently greater wall thickening. The various methods of defining myocardial borders, the cross-sectional views selected for analysis, and the application of different reference methods for analysis constitute sources of the discrepancies reported in the literature for measurements of regional wall motion. Whereas the eye can integrate the factors of image quality, cardiac rotation, translation, and wall thickening in the 2D image of a beating heart to provide a qualitative interpretation, it has proven to be a very difficult task to accomplish the same thing in quantitative analysis. The importance of achieving quantitative, and preferably on-line, assessment of dynamic cardiac function, however, cannot be over-estimated.

REFERENCES

1. Herman MV, Hemle RA, Klein MD, Jorlin R: Localized disorders in myocardial contraction: asynergy and its role in congestive heart failure. N Engl J Med 277:222–232, 1967.
2. Greenbaum RA, Ho Sy, Gibson DE, Becker AE, Anderson RH: Left ventricular fibre architecture in man. Br Heart J 45:248–263, 1981.
3. Kong Y, Morris JJ, McIntosh HD: Assessment of regional myocardial performance from biplane coronary cineangiograms. Am J Cardiol 27:529–537, 1971.
4. Liedke JA, Gault JH, Leman DR, Blumenthal MS: Geometry of left ventricular contraction in the systolic click syndrome. Circulation 47:27–35, 1973.
5. Shapiro E, Marier DL, St. John Sutton ME, Gibson DE: Regional nonuniformity of wall dynamics in normal left ventricle. Br Heart J 45:264–270, 1981.
6. Haendchen RV, Wyatt HL, Maurer J, Zwehl W, Baer M, Meerbaum S, Corday E: Quantitation of regional cardiac function by two-dimensional echocardiography. I. Patterns of contraction in the normal left ventricle. Circulation 67:1234–1245, 1983.
7. Leighton RF, Wilt SM, Lewis RP: Detection of hypokinesis by a quantitative analysis of left ventricular cineangiograms. Circulation 50:121–127, 1974.
8. Le Winter MM, Kent RS, Kroener JM, Caren TW, Covell JW: Regional differences in myocardial performance in the left ventricle of the dog. Circ Res 37:191–199, 1975.
9. Marcus ML, Kerber RE, Ehrhardt J, Abboud FM: Three dimensional geometry of acutely ischemic myocardium. Circulation 52:254–263, 1975.
10. Klausner SC, Tarlton JB, Bulawa WF, Jeppson GM, Jensen RL, Clayton PD: Quantitative analysis of segmental wall motion throughout systole and diastole in the normal human left ventricle. Circulation 65:580–590, 1982.
11. Ruttley MS, Adams DF, Cohn PF, Abrams HL: Shape and volume changes during "isovolumic relaxation" in normal and asynergic ventricles. Circulation 50:306–316, 1974.
12. Altieri PI, Wilt SM, Leighton RF: Left ventricular wall motion during the isovolume relaxation period. Circulation 48:499–505, 1973.
13. Gibson DG, Prewitt TA, Brown DJ: Analysis of left ventricular wall movement during isovolumic relaxation and its relation to coronary artery disease. Br Heart J 38:1010–1019, 1978.

14. Assad-Morell JL, Tajik AJ, Giuliani ER: Echocardiographic analysis of the ventricular septum. Prog Cardiovasc Dis 17:219–237, 1974.
15. McDonald IG: Echocardiographic demonstration of abnormal motion of the interventricular septum in left bundle branch block. Circulation 48:272–280, 1973.
16. King JF, DeMaria AN, Bonanno JA, et al: The temporal sequence of myocardial contraction in bundle branch block determined by echocardiography [abstr]. Circulation [Suppl 4] 48:127, 1973.
17. Dillon JC, Chang S, Feigenbaum H: Echocardiographic manifestations of left bundle branch block [abstr]. Circulation [Suppl 4] 49:126, 1973.
18. Abbasi AS, Eber LM, MacAlpin RN, et al: Paradoxical motion of interventricular septum in left bundle branch block. Circulation 49:423–427, 1974.
19. Holman BL, Wynne J, Idoine J, Neill J: Disruption in the temporal sequency of regional ventricular contraction. I. Characteristics and incidence in coronary artery disease. Circulation 61:1075–1083, 1980.
20. Jacobs JJ, Feigenbaum H, Corya BC: Detection of left ventricular asynergy by echocardiography. Circulation 48:263–271, 1973.
21. Schnittger T, Fitzgerald PJ, Daughters GT, Ingels NB, Kantrowitz NE, Schwartzkopf A, Mead CW, Popp RL: Limitations of comparing left ventricular volumes by two-dimensional echocardiography, myocardial markers and cineangiography. Am J Cardiol 50:512–519, 1982.
22. Rankin JS, McHale PA, Arentzen CE, Ling D, Greenfield JC, Anderson RW: Three dimensional dynamic geometry of the left ventricle in the conscious dog. Circ Res 39:304–313, 1976.
23. Cooper RH, O'Rourke RA, Karliner JS, Peterson KL, Leopold JR: Comparison of ultrasound and cineangiographic measurements of the mean rate of circumferential fiber shortening in man. Circulation 46:914–923, 1972.
24. Sahn DJ, Deely WJ, Hagan AD, Friedman WF: Echocardiographic assessment of left ventricular performance in normal newborns. Circulation 49:232–236, 1974.
25. Gutgesell HP, Paquet M, Duff DF, McNamara DG: Evaluation of left ventricular size and function by echocardiography: results in normal children. Circulation 56:457–462, 1977.
26. Nixon JV, Murray RG, Leonard PD, Mitchell JH, Blomqirst CG: Effect of large variations in preload on left ventricular performance characteristics in normal subjects. Circulation 65:698–703, 1982.
27. Quinones MA, Mokotoff DM, Nouri S, Winters WL, Miller RR: Noninvasive quantification of left ventricular wall stress: validation of method and application to assessment of chronic pressure overload. Am J Cardiol 45:782–790, 1980.
28. Reichek N, Wilson J, St. John Sutton M, Plappert TA, Goldberg S, Hirshfeld JW: Noninvasive determination of left ventricular end-systolic stress: validation of the method and initial application. Circulation 65:99–108, 1982.
29. Strauer BE: Myocardial oxygen consumption in chronic heart disease: role of wall stress, hypertrophy and coronary reserve. Am J Cardiol 44:730–740, 1979.
30. Sagawa K: The ventricular pressure–volume diagram revisited. Circ Res 43:677–687, 1978.
31. Suga H, Sagawa K: Instantaneous pressure–volume relationships and their ratio in the excised, supported canine left ventricle. Circ Res 35:117–126, 1974.
32. Suga H, Sagawa K, Kostiuk DP: Controls of ventricular contractility assessed by pressure–volume ratio E_{max}. Cardiovasc Res 10:582–592, 1976.
33. Hoffman BF, Bassett AL, Bartelstone HJ: Some mechanical properties of isolated mammalian cardiac muscle. Circ Res 23:291–312, 1968.
34. Lakatta EG, Lappe DL: Diastolic scattered light fluctuation, resting force and twitch force in mammalian cardiac muscle. J Physiol (Lon) 315:369–394, 1981.

35. Lappe DL, Lakatta EG: Intensity fluctuation spectroscopy monitors contractile activation in "resting" cardiac muscle. Science 297:1369–1371, 1980.

36. Stein PD, Sabbah HN, Marzilli M, Blick EF: Comparison of the distribution of intramyocardial pressure across the canine left ventricular wall in the beating heart during diastole and in the arrested heart: evidence of epicardial muscle tone during diastole. Circ Res 47:258–267, 1980.

37. Diamond G, Forrester JS: Effect of coronary artery disease and acute myocardial infarction on left ventricular compliance in man. Circulation 45:11–19, 1972.

39. Dodek A, Kassebaum DG, Bristow JD: Pulmonary edema in coronary artery disease without cardiomegaly: paradox of the stiff heart. N Engl J Med 286:1347–1350, 1972.

39. Gibson DG, Prewitt TA, Brown DJ: Analysis of left ventricular wall movement during isovolumic relaxation and its relation to coronary artery disease. Br Heart J 38:1010–1019, 1976.

40. Gibson DG, Doran JH, Traill TA, Brown DJ: Regional abnormalities of left ventricular wall movement during isovolumic relaxation in patients with ischemic heart disease. Eur J Cardiol [Suppl] 7:251–264, 1978.

41. Barry WH, Brooker JZ, Alderman EH, Harrison DC: Changes in diastolic stiffness and one of the left ventricle during angina pectoris. Circulation 49:255–263, 1974.

42. Dwyer EM: Left ventricular pressure–volume alterations and regional disorders of contraction during myocardial ischemia induced by atrial pacing. Circulation 42:1111–1122, 1970.

43. Flessas AP, Connelly GP, Handa S, Tilney CR, Kloster CK, Rimmer RH Jr, Keefe JF, Klein MD, Ryan TH: Effects of isometric exercise on the end-diastolic pressure, volumes and function of the left ventricle in man. Circulation 53:839–847, 1976.

44. Mann T, Brodie BR, Grossman W, McLaurin LP: Effect of angina on the left ventricular diastolic pressure–volume relationship. Circulation 55:761–766, 1977.

45. Bourdillon PD, Lorell BH, Mirsky I, Paulus WJ, Wynne T, Grossman W: Increased regional myocardial stiffness of the left ventricle during pacing-induced angina in man. Circulation 67:316–323, 1983.

46. Grossman W, Barry WH: Diastolic pressure–volume relations in the diseased heart. Fed Proc 39:148–155, 1980.

47. Sheehan FH, Dodge HT, Bolson EL, Hok-Wai W, Caputo GR, Stewart DK: Value of partial ejection fraction, volume increment, and regional wall motion in identifying patients with clinically significant coronary artery disease. Circulation 68:756–762, 1983.

48. Sheehan FH, Stewart DK, Dodge HT, Smitten S, Bolson EL, Brown BG: Variability in the measurement of regional left ventricular wall motion from contrast angiograms. Circulation 68:550–559, 1983.

49. Field BJ, Russell RD Jr, Dowling JT, Rackley CE: Regional left ventricular performance in the year following myocardial infarction. Circulation 46:679–689, 1972.

50. Gelberg HF, Brundage BH, Clantz S, Parmley WW: Quantitative left ventricular well motion analysis: a comparison of area, chord and radial methods. Circulation 59:991–1000, 1979.

51. Karsch KR, Lamm U, Blanke H, Pentrop KP: Comparison of nineteen quantitative models for assessment of localized left ventricular wall motion abnormalities. Clin Cardiol 3:124–128, 1980.

52. Moynihan PF, Parish AF, Feldman CL: Quantitative detection of regional left ventricular contraction abnormalities by two-dimensional echocardiography. Circulation 63:752–760, 1981.

53. Schnittger I, Fitzgerald PJ, Jordon EP, Alderman EL, Popp RL: Computerized quantitative analysis of left ventricular wall motion by two-dimensional echocardiography. Circulation 70:242–254, 1984.
54. Parisi AF, Moynihan PF, Folland ED, Feldman CL: Quantitative detection of regional left ventricular contraction abnormalities by two-dimensional echocardiography. II. Accuracy in coronary artery disease. Circulation 63:761–767, 1981.
55. Grube E, Hanisch H, Neumann J, Simon H: Quantitative evaluation of LV-wall motion by two-dimensional echocardiography (2-DE) [abstr]. J Am Coll Cardiol 1:581, 1983.
56. Pandian NG, Kerber RE: Two-dimensional echocardiography in experimental coronary stenosis. I. Sensitivity and specificity in detecting transient myocardial dyskinesis: comparison with sonomicrometers. Circulation 63:597–602, 1982.
57. McDonald IG, Geigenbaum H, Chang S: Analysis of left ventricular wall motion by reflected ultrasound. Circulation 46:14–25, 1972.
58. Troy BL, Pombo J, Rackley CE: Measurement of left ventricular wall thickness and mass by echocardiography. Circulation 45:602–611, 1972.
59. Gaasch WH, Andrias CW, Levine HF: Chronic aortic regurgitation: the effect of aortic valve replacement on left ventricular volume, mass and function. Circulation 58:825–836, 1978.
60. Feigel EO, Fry DL: Myocardial mural thickness during the cardiac cycle. Circ Res 14:541–545, 1964.
61. Mitchell JH, Widenthal K, Mullins CB: Geometrical studies of the left ventricle using biplane cinefluorography. Fed Proc 28:1334–1343, 1969.
62. Sasayama I, Franklin D, Ross J, Kemper WS, McKown D: Dynamic changes on left ventricular wall thickness and their use in analyzing cardiac function in the conscious dog. Am J Cardiol 38:870–879, 1976.
63. Feneley MP, Hickie JB: Validity of echocardiographic determination of left ventricular systolic wall thickening. Circulation 70:226–232, 1984.
64. Wyatt HL, Haendchen RV, Meerbaum S, Corday E: Assessment of quantitative methods for 2-dimensional echocardiography. Am J Cardiol 52:396–401, 1983.

6. DOPPLER ECHOCARDIOGRAPHY

As ultrasound technology has developed into a practical method for imaging cardiac structures, the incorporation of another technique using ultrasound, for the measurement of blood flow and direction, has followed naturally. Doppler echocardiography was first reported by Satumora [1] and is widely available as an adjunctive diagnostic procedure with echocardiography. With advancing computer technology, Doppler echocardiography is providing more and more clinical information, all in a noninvasive procedure.

The traditional example of the Doppler effect is that of the abrupt change in tone of the train whistle as the train speeds by. As the train approaches, the sound waves traveling toward us from the whistle are compressed so that the frequency or pitch of the sound appears higher than if the whistle were stationary. At the instant the train passes and moves away from us, the sound becomes lower in pitch, or frequency. Thus, the Doppler effect refers to the frequency shift that occurs when the distance between the sound source and its reception is changing. The same phenomenon applies to frequencies in the inaudible range, such as ultrasound, reflected from a moving object. This allows for the identification of blood flow, when ultrasound from a stationary transducer is transmitted to, and reflected by, red blood cells [2]. The reflected ultrasound received by the transducer has undergone a frequency shift since it was transmitted. The frequency shift is determined by the formula:

$$\Delta F = \frac{2f_1 v \cos \theta}{C} \tag{1}$$

where ΔF = the difference between transmitted and received frequencies, f_1 = the transmitted frequency, v = blood velocity, C = speed of sound in the tissue ($1540\,\mathrm{m\,s^{-1}}$), and θ is the intercept angle between the axis of the blood flow and the ultrasound beam.

The two major variables influencing the Doppler frequency shift are the intercept angle and the blood flow velocity. The maximum Doppler frequency shift for any blood flow velocity will occur when the angle is zero degrees.

For the determination of blood flow velocity, equation 1 becomes:

$$v = \frac{\Delta F \cdot C}{2f_1 \cdot \cos \theta} \tag{2}$$

In order to reduce the angle theta to zero, and measure blood flow accurately, the transducer must be positioned so as to orient the ultrasound beam as nearly parallel to the blood flow as possible. Normally, blood flow in the heart and great vessels can be considered as laminar; thus, red blood cells in the bloodstream are moving at the same speed and in the same direction, except near the walls of the vessel or chamber where flow is slightly slower, and their Doppler frequency shifts are similar. Disorganized, turbulent flow, as occurs around stenotic valves or with intracardiac shunts, does not have a measurable flow velocity by Doppler, since red blood cells are moving at different speeds, in different directions.

CONTINUOUS AND PULSED DOPPLER

Two principal methods of ultrasound transmission have been employed to take advantage of the Doppler effect. Transducers have been designed to emit either a continuous wave of ultrasound or intermittent pulses. With pulsed Doppler, the time interval between pulse emission and reception of the reflected wave allows for the localization of the area from which the ultrasound is reflected. Thus, on the accompanying echocardiographic image, a specific Doppler frequency shift can be traced to its geographic origin within the cardiac chamber or blood vessel. This site represents the sample volume of the ultrasound beam. The sample volume can be selected at will for the detection and measurement of blood flow in various parts of the heart as indicated on an echocardiographic image. Pulsed Doppler, therefore, offers some advantage for the localization of a measured blood flow. However, accurate recording of high-frequency Doppler shifts common with high-velocity blood flow is limited by the relatively low sampling rate imposed by the pulse repetition frequency. This pulse repetition frequency is limited by the time that must be allowed between pulses for the ultrasound to travel to and from the target. Further, this same time constraint limits the depth of field that can be examined, since the ultrasound pulse will take longer to travel to and from a target situated far from the transducer. Thus, the higher the pulse repetition frequency is set, the higher the maximum blood flow velocity detectable, but the use of a high pulse repetition frequency limits the depth of field that can be examined.

Continuous wave Doppler allows a high sampling rate, and is well suited for the assessment of high-velocity blood flows, but it does not permit localization of the Doppler frequency shift. "High pulse repetition frequency Doppler" is a technique designed to incorporate the advantages of both continuous wave and pulsed Doppler systems; the Doppler sampling rate is increased by integer multiples, with a corresponding increase in the number of sampling volumes along the ultrasound beam. This permits assessment of high-velocity blood flows, and provides some localization capability.

QUANTITATION OF FLOW

The quantitation of blood flow requires a measurement of volume, and for this purpose echocardiographic data is combined with Doppler information. Flow (volume) = flow velocity ($cm \cdot s^{-1}$) × duration of flow (s) × cross-sectional area of the vessel or valve orifice through which the blood flows (cm^2). The product of average flow velocity and duration is provided by the area under the curve of the flow velocity curve. This calculation, however, requires that a number of assumptions are made: the great vessels, or valvular orifices, are assumed to be circular; flow velocity and cross sectional area are assumed to be derived from the same place; blood flow is assumed to be laminar with a blunt velocity profile; and flow is assumed to fill the measured cross-sectional area completely.

Doppler information is processed to provide both auditory and graphic outputs. The auditory signal delivers a spectrum of sound corresponding to the spectrum of ultrasound frequencies received from the moving red blood cells. Laminar flow produces musical, smooth sounds, whereas turbulent flow results in noisy, harsh sounds. With some experience, the listener can derive some useful information, but, clearly, the auditory signal is a qualitative one. Graphic output, however, is presented as a time interval histogram in which a pattern of dots printed on a strip chart recording denotes the direction and velocity of flow. Flow toward the transducer is shown as a positive deflection, and flow away from the transducer as a negative deflection. Zero flow therefore is represented at baseline. This format lends itself for quantitative analysis by computer techniques. With the ability to derive quantitative information, Doppler echocardiography has found immediate application in the measurement of cardiac output, or flow through the aorta.

Magnin and coworkers [3] measured flow volumes with a pulsed Doppler flowmeter in combination with a phased array imaging system both in vitro and in patients undergoing cardiac catheterization. The 2D imaging system was used to obtain the diameter of the orifice through which the flow occurred, and the range and angle of the Doppler sample volume were determined by superimposition of a cursor line on the 2D image. In vitro validation of this method was done by measuring continuous flow through tubing in water tank (figure 6-1). The results correlated very well with measured flow corresponding to a physiologic range of 3–12 l/min ($r = 0.99$). With pulsatile flow in this model (figure 6-2), the correlation coefficient was slightly lower ($r = 0.86$). The clinical evaluation of the system in 11 patients, comparing cardiac output measurements with Doppler and Fick methods, yielded a correlation coefficient of 0.83. In this small number of patients, there was also a significant offset from zero at the origin of the curve (figure 6-3).

Since the noninvasive assessment of cardiac output is immediately attractive for critical care, particularly intraoperatively, a number of investigators have evaluated continuous wave Doppler for this purpose, using an esophageal transducer to measure cardiac output in the ascending or descending aorta.

All showed that cardiac output can be measured easily and reliably with this technique, correlating well with simultaneous thermodilution cardiac output determinations. Payen and coworkers [4] have reported a correlation coefficient of 0.96 in a study of 26 intensive care patients using both of these methods. Small systems to continuously measure cardiac output transesophageally are now commercially available. In addition to assessment of global cardiac flow, or output,

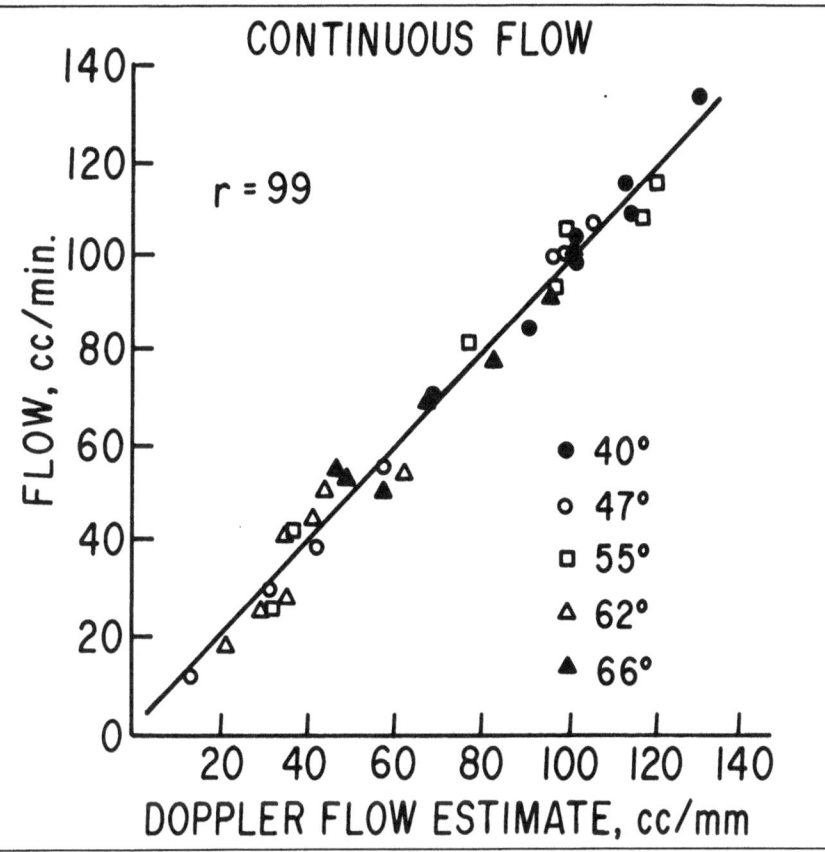

Figure 6-1. Relationship between continuous flow measured using a stopwatch and a graduated cylinder and a Doppler phased array system Reproduced with permission from Magnin et al. [3].

Doppler finds application for the evaluation of stenosis and regurgitation occurring at or near the valves, and for shunts, e.g., atrial septal defects, ventricular septal defects, patent ductus arteriosus.

AORTIC VALVULAR FLOW

The aortic valve lies in a relatively anterior position within the heart and flow through it is directed anteriorly and superiorly. Thus, flow is detected quite readily using transthoracic Doppler, with the transducer placed at a high parasternal location. Flow then appears directed toward the transducer unless there is regurgitation into the left ventricle, away from the transducer. With aortic stenosis, producing a high-velocity jet and some turbulence, the graphic display shows systolic dot scatter, or spectral broadening, as ultrasound waves are

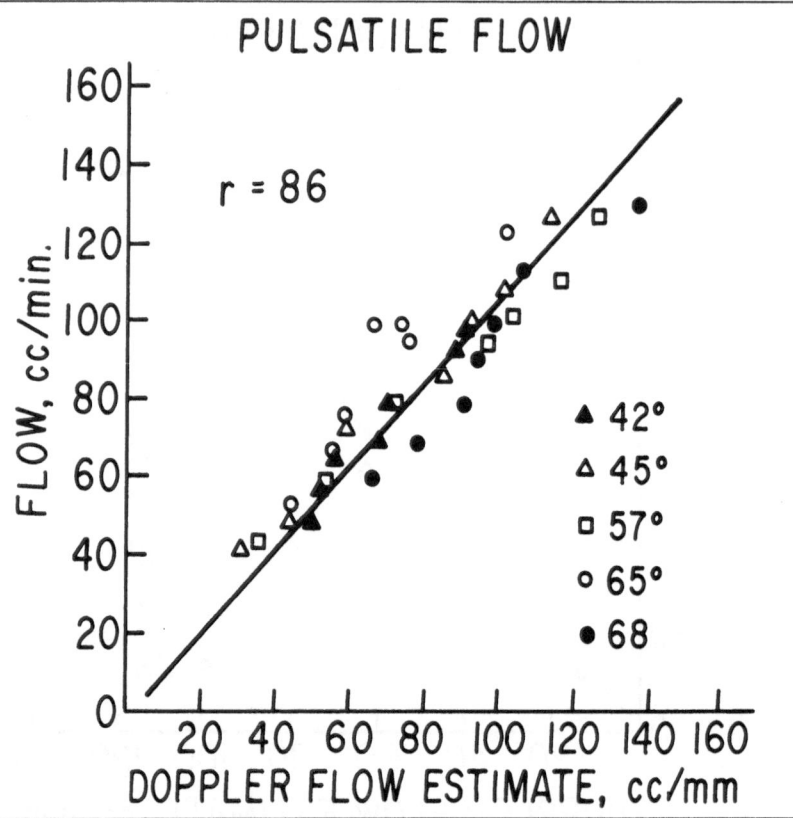

Figure 6-2. Relationship between pulsatile flow measured using a stopwatch and a graduated cylinder and a Doppler phased array system. Reproduced with permission form Magnin et al. [3].

reflected from red cells in the turbulent stream. The maximum flow velocity in the poststenotic turbulent jet permits an estimation of the pressure gradient across the valve, using a modified Bernoulli equation:

$$\Delta P = 4(V_{max})^2$$

MITRAL VALVULAR FLOW

The mitral valve lies posterior in the heart, close to the esophagus, but far from the chest wall. Flow through the valve is directed inferiorly and anteriorly from the left atrium into the left ventricle, and the placement of a transducer emitting ultrasound in a direction parallel to this flow is difficult from the chest wall. In the parasternal position, ultrasound is emitted almost perpendicular to the flow and, if it is

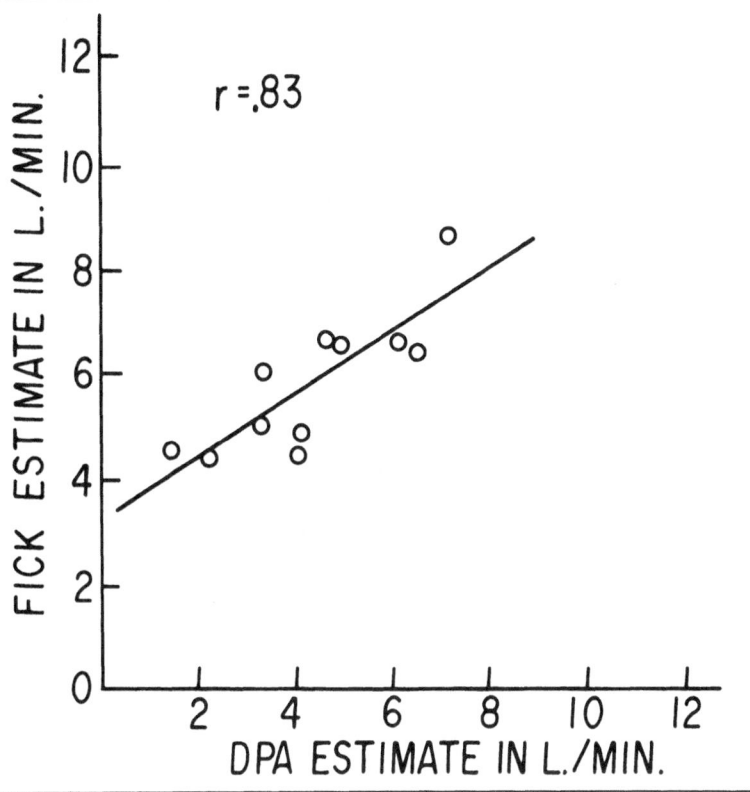

Figure 6-3. Cardiac output by Fick estimate in 11 patients compared with a Doppler phased array system estimate of cardiac output. Reproduced with permission from Magnin et al. [3].

placed at the left side of the chest at the cardiac apex, there is a relatively large distance between the transducer and the mitral valve, so that high pulse repetition frequencies cannot be used. Flow, normally occurring only in diastole, is directed toward the apical transducer with an early diastolic peak being followed by a period of diastasis and then a late peak caused by atrial contraction. During systole, there should be no signals, with no flow from the ventricle into the atrium. With mitral stenosis, diastolic flow is prolonged and appears turbulent; with regurgitation, there is turbulent flow away from the transducer during systole.

Because of the difficulty with a transthoracic approach, some investigators [5, 6] have used an esophageal transducer. Schluter and coworkers [6] evaluated six patients with competent mitral valves and 12 patients with angiographically proven mild-to-moderate mitral regurgitation. The transesophageal approach detected regurgitation in 100% of cases, whereas the transthoracic approach was successful in only 58%. The closer position of the esophageal transducer provided high-quality recordings, and allowed the ultrasound beam to be emitted in a direction parallel to the blood flow. Since a high pulse repetition frequency could be used by virtue of the proximity of the transducer to the mitral valve, the regurgitant jets could be localized by left atrial scanning.

INTRACARDIAC SHUNTS

With Doppler echocardiography, intracardiac shunts can be detected by recording turbulence downstream from the lesion, and by selecting a sample volume within the observed defect to confirm the presence of blood flow through it. For example, turbulence from a ventricular septal defect can be detected in the right ventricular outflow tract. The interventricular septum can then be "explored" with ultrasound to define the point at which abnormal flow signals are most obvious. A sample volume can then be "threaded" through the defect to confirm the presence of abnormal flow.

2D DOPPLER COLOR FLOW MAPPING

Until very recently, Doppler technology has been limited to the techniques described above. Thus, real-time measurement of intracardiac blood flows has been restricted to a single point at any one time. To "map" the entire intracardiac blood flow, there must be information from an infinite number of points at the same time. This kind of Doppler information is now becoming available with the advent of color flow mapping. This system uses pulsed Doppler in combination with a 2D echocardiograph and employs a wide-angle phased array transducer. Current designs use a frequency of 2.5 MHz and a pulse repetition frequency of 4 kHz, which allows for a depth of field of 18 cm. Each 2D cross-sectional image is composed of echoes generated by ultrasound reflected from 32 elements each emitting eight pulses in succession. One sector scan takes 66 ms to complete. The reflected ultrasound waves are separated electronically into two parts: high-amplitude components reflected from cardiac structures provide the cardiac image, and low-amplitude waves representing reflected echoes from moving red blood cells provide blood flow information. Cardiac structures are displayed in a monochrome mode whereas blood flow and direction are presented in a color-coded format at the rate of 15 frames per second in real time. Blood flow toward the transducer is displayed as red, and blood flow away from the transducer appears blue. Magnitude of flow is indicated by the brightness of color, and turbulence, detected as variance of blood velocity within a sample volume, is represented by a quantity of green added according to the amount of velocity variance. Thus, the blood flow is characterized according to its direction, magnitude, and turbulence by color, presented in real time directly on the 2D cardiac image, by simultaneously sampling muliple areas within the cardiac chambers. In fact, there is a slight delay of 2 ms in the processing of this information as signals are received and integrated from 16,000 points comprising the 2D image, 500 points along each of the 32 ultrasound beams from the transducer [7].

Qualitatively, color flow mapping provides a rapid orientation to the presence and location of small atrial and ventricular septal defects that might be missed with conventional Doppler echocardiography. It also identifies the occurrence of multiple ventricular septal defects often not appreciated by the older diagnostic methods [8]. Miyatake and coworkers [7] reported its use for the rapid identification of valvular insufficiency, but noted some apparent signal noise problems and difficulty arising from the limited depth of field permitted with the system. Such difficulties may be overcome with the advent of transesophageal color flow mapping for the same reasons that make conventional echocardiographic images of the posterior structures superior with an esophageal transducer. The potential applications in complex congenital heart disease are considerable, both for the cardiologist and the anesthesiologist.

REFERENCES

1. Satumora S: Ultrasonic Doppler method for the inspection of cardiac functions. J Acoust Soc Am 29:1181–1185, 1957.
2. Franklin DL, Schlegel W, Rushmer RF: Blood flow measured by Doppler frequency shift backscattered sound. Science 134:564–565, 1961.
3. Magnin PA, Stewart JA, Myers S, Von Ramm O, Kisslo JA: Combined Doppler and phased-array echocardiographic estimation of cardiac output. Circulation 63:388–392, 1981.
4. Payen D, Fidgeu J, Levy B: Pulsed Doppler cardiac output and left ventricular pumping ability measurements during artificial ventilation [abstr]. Anesthesiology 61:A170, 1984.
5. Hisanaga K, Hisanaga A, Ichie J, Nishimura K, Hibi N, Fukui Y, Kambe T: Transesophageal pulsed Doppler echocardiography. Lancet 1:53–54, 1979.
6. Schlüter M, Langenstein BA, Hanrath P, Kremer P, Bleifeld W: Assessment of transesophageal pulsed Doppler echocardiography in the detection of mitral regurgitation. Circulation 66:784–789, 1982.

7. Miyatake K, Okamoto M, Kinoshita N, Trumi S, Owa M, Takao S, Sakakibara H, Nimura Y: Clinical applications of a new type of real-time two-dimensional Doppler flow imaging system. Am J Cardiol 54:857–868, 1985.
8. Sahn DJ, Swensson RE, Valdez-Cruz LM, Scagnelli S, Main J: Two-dimensional color flow mapping for evaluation of ventricular septal defect shunts: a new diagnostic modality [abstr]. Circulation [Suppl 2] 70:II-364, 1984.

INDEX